Testimonials for *Recover y*

There are several full testimon[i]   are
some synopses:

"After suffering with fatigue for 20 years and diagnosed with ME 13 years ago, this was the last big step in helping me to wellness. I had never before got over the pain in my legs when I did even the lightest exercise and I would take months to recover. I am now able to run, walk up stairs and do things without pain and debilitating tiredness..." Helen, Hertfordshire

"Your book is wonderful - it takes us on a journey of discovery, following the path to good health, removing stuck energy and making us aware of how powerful our subconscious mind is. Thank you for helping me recover my energy." Katherine, Buckinghamshire

"This book will bring hope and relief to many people. Olive has a wonderful gift and passion for taking what could be complicated ideas and processes and making them easily accessible to everyone. Reading it will trigger conscious changes for vitality, and also teach your unconscious mind how to take better care of your body and your health. Many, many people will experience more health and vitality as a result of this book." Art Giser, San Francisco

"Olive was a enormous help with our 14 year old daughter who was suffering from ME like symptoms. Thanks to Olive she has made a full recovery, in just a few weeks, after 5 months off school. Highly recommended." David, Sussex

"At last, a self-help book supplying your very own personal support team who encourage and guide you to find your own personal way to wellness! Thanks Olive, not only has *Recovery Your Energy* given me and my family new & effective tools, I wish my children had been able to read it when they were even younger. Your style of writing makes the invaluable information accessible to any age reader. Essential family reading to help prevent poor health!" Sue, the Netherlands

RECOVER YOUR

ENERGY

By

OLIVE HICKMOTT

www.recoveryourenergy.co.uk

Published by

MX Publishing

A New Perspectives Book

**For more information about the book take a look at:
www.recoveryourenergy.co.uk and for the associated health
and wellness practice www.empoweringhealth.co.uk**

ISBN13 9781904312574

First published in 2009
© Copyright 2009
Olive Hickmott

Although every effort has been made to assure the accuracy of the information contained in this guide as of the date of publication, nothing herein should be construed as giving specific treatment advice. In addition, the application of the techniques to specific circumstances can present complex issues that are beyond the scope of this guide. This publication is intended to provide general information pertaining to developing these skills.

Published in the UK by MX Publishing, 335, Princess Park Manor, Royal Drive, London, N11 3GX
www.mxpublishing.co.uk

Dedication

I would like to dedicate this book to all those children and adults overwhelmed by fatigue, often at a very early age, and often for a very long time indeed. This book is for you and others like you, a straightforward and simple path to lead you back to where you want to be and nurture you in the process.

"THIS BOOK WILL ENERGISE YOU"

About the author

My name is **Olive Hickmott and** I have a passion for helping those with chronic illness and/or learning difficulties set, achieve and surpass their goals.

I'm lucky enough to be doing what I consider the best job in the world. I'm an inveterate puzzle-solver and health challenges and what causes them can be the greatest puzzles of all, for an individual to unravel. Luckily, so often the key lies within us, we have such fabulous self-healing skills, it's just a question of learning how to access them.

I am an NLP Master Practitioner, EnergeticNLP Practitioner, a Thought Pattern Management Master Practitioner and a Certified Coach.

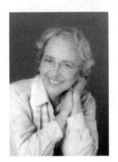 Utilising all my training I work with individuals and groups, enabling personal growth in all aspects of their lives. It's a great privilege to be there at moments when individuals first grasp the interlinking of mind, body and spirit and get their first glimpses of what they can achieve.

I also work within businesses to improve the well-being of both staff and directors, improving their communication and relationships and ultimately the profitability that results from a smoother running company.

I exited my own corporate life as an Engineering Director in 1990 and founded my own business. I am a Director of the Hickmott Partnership.

I focus on primary research working with those people who know their specific health challenges well. They have helped me develop and articulate the *New Perspectives* approach to energetic well-being and without their valuable assistance, this would not have been possible.

NEW PERSPECTIVES

With every new day you have a choice; a choice to do things differently.

If you choose the same actions as yesterday, you will get the same results - try another way.

"The world is full of obvious things which nobody by any chance ever observes"
Sherlock Holmes

Previous New Perspectives books:
Seeing Spells Achieving
You too can 'do' health!

Acknowledgements

There are many people I wish to thank for their help and influence in writing this book. In particular:

Art Giser, creator of EnergeticNLP, without whose teaching and generosity, none of this would have been possible. (www.energeticNLP.com)

Ian McDermott, Robert Dilts, Tim Hallbom and Suzi Smith for their ideas and teaching that have contributed much to my ability as a Health Coach and an author.

Peter King, who has inspired so many to realise that with curiosity major changes become possible and the impossible melts away.

Jill Southgate, my tireless editor, those who volunteered to review this book from their different perspectives and Marilyn Messik for polishing my words.

Steve Emecz, my publisher at mxpublishing, whose expert advice for the project has been so valuable.

Penny Perry for her fabulous illustrations; she has the great skill to be able to bring characters in the book to life on the page.

Diana Kingham who contributed the appendix to match some of the medical knowledge to the energetic and emotional world in which I practice.

And finally to thank my family who not only read parts of the script but challenged my thinking and above all supported me throughout the project.

Preface

It's puzzling, isn't it? With so much energy throughout nature, how can anyone possibly feel fatigued? Why is fatigue a daily experience for millions of people? Why for many of them is it the dominant experience of their lives?[1]

THIS BOOK WILL ENERGISE YOU. You'll learn about your own personal energy system and how, by "setting it to wellness" you can have all the energy you want. You'll learn, through a simple tale how to tap into the amazing power of *your* mind with energy enhanced NLP (EnergeticNLP); recognise how your thoughts negatively or positively affect your energy and develop skills that will gain you optimum health, wellness and vitality.

Storytellers through the ages and psychologists more recently, are in agreement that stories have direct access to the healing part of the mind. In escaping into a simple story your mind and body can pick up the messages they need and you'll have started that trip back to wellness.

Journeying through this book will enable you to mobilise your own internal **team** to recover your energy effectively. I use a light-hearted approach but with a complete awareness of the profound emotional, physical and energetic manifestations we are dealing with.

Recover your energy is designed and written for those of you seeking increased energy and restored vitality: whether you have occasional exhaustion or have been running on empty for some time and have

---

[1] Deepak Chopra, Boundless Energy, Page 2

developed major fatigue. We've all of course experienced those feelings of extreme fatigue, for example, flu-ridden we can't even muster up enough energy to reach for a glass of water. With extreme fatigue this is an ongoing feeling, the consistency of which saps you even further.

Perhaps you have been labelled as having Myalgic Encephalomyelitis (ME), Chronic Fatigue Syndrome (CFS), Seasonal Affective Disorder(SAD), Glandular Fever, Post-viral Syndrome (CFS). Unfortunately diagnosis doesn't run hand in hand with cure.

In common with those who have illnesses such as Multiple Sclerosis (MS), Cancer or Parkinson's you may be experiencing tremendous energy dips – you feel low on energy, mindless with fatigue and are often suffering associated shooting or continual pain – this is *not* just normal tiredness.

Unsurprisingly, people who have chronic fatigue often know little about how their own personal energy *works*. My belief, clearly demonstrated by work with my clients, is that simple techniques of energy hygiene, can hugely increase vitality. This book is the torch that can light your path to recovery!

We've all met uncomfortably negative people in our time. Those who unload a bucketful of woes and leave you feeling completely drained - the result of picking up a large dose of their negative energy. And then there are those who trigger intense emotion in you, maybe anger, guilt or frustration which means you're then flooding your system with your own stored up negative energy. All of this negativity *blows your fuses* leaving you empty and tired.

As you move further into the book you'll find other factors that also have this unfortunate effect – you'll also learn how to actively counteract this and grab that energy back.

Should you have concerns that you are developing fatigue it's important to accept that it happens gradually and insidiously, over time and that "an ounce of prevention is worth a pound of cure!" By utilising what this book has to offer you'll be able to take up tools and adopt techniques that will halt your energy seepage *before* it becomes severe and restore you to normal balance.

We really can't imagine not brushing our teeth or washing ourselves on a daily basis. However, exactly like your physical body, your energy system gets clogged and grubby with other people's negative energy or by the triggering of your own negative emotions. EnergeticNLP which underpins this story, may be considered at one level to be the personal hygiene tool for the energy system. Techniques used are simple guided imagery and the best news is there's no special equipment needed, other than an open mind. More advanced techniques of EnergeticNLP, although not covered in this book, are those that enable a practitioner to assist you in person or over the phone to identify and shift energy blocks. These methods can be used to suit your individual lifestyle – now what could be simpler or easier to implement?

It's my sincere hope you'll find something to smile about in the energy-managing approach I've taken and never underestimate the healing power of humour, *the funnier you find things, the faster your progress will be.*

So park any judgemental feelings firmly on the side lines and let your imaginative brain take charge of the images you find in the story. Fatigue is no respecter of age, sex or social standing and is paradoxically very often seen in those who have been the most active, vibrant and energetic throughout their lives. Even youngsters who develop fatigue, can find this book easily digestible.

In my years of work with chronic fatigue sufferers and those experiencing debilitating pains, I've often noted a series of triggers that set the fatigue ball in motion. These are often linked to a major life change (new school, university, marriage, divorce, bereavement) that is stressful to that particular individual. If a viral infection hits the body at the same time as it's already coping with greater than normal levels of stress stirred up by change, the energy system can take such a hit, that recovery is not easy.

Because we're all different, some of us are more energy sensitive than others. We can be affected by other people's energy and by our surroundings as well as by what's going on in our own internal systems. If this barrage continues over a long period of time, other health challenges can also appear.

Recover your energy is intended to enhance conventional or complementary medicine, not replace it. It empowers you to take action, using the resources you already possess but may not have recognised, to positively affect your health and speed recovery. If you would like to read more of the medical knowledge and existing approaches to the treatment of fatigue take a look at Appendix 1.

The New Perspectives project

I started the New Perspectives project to help people with fatigue to recover their energy using the tools of Neuro-linguistic Programming (NLP) and EnergeticNLP. Each of my clients knew they were lacking energy and wanted to find how to rediscover it.

I learned such a lot from clients I helped during this project, in effect *they* taught *me* how best to help them. The great results that emerged from this work have always been freely shared with other practitioners, so we can further refine the tools to help those suffering from symptoms of fatigue. My philosophy is not to keep control of these processes but to open them up to everyone as a service to health. During the project I have seen many people who have been exposed to negative energy almost from birth. The effect of this often doesn't show itself until around the age of 20 although even children, as young as 6, have been found to exhibit symptoms.

I wrote this book because:

- √ I wanted to provide an invaluable resource for those I meet who are suffering with fatigue and associated pain.

- √ I wanted to arm those people who are *new* to fatigue with tools they can use before they are really ill. In essence, "head the illness off at the pass!"

- √ I felt it was so important to find a way of reaching the millions fatigued or diagnosed as such, so they can avoid long-term illness.

- √ I have personally experienced exactly what fatigue and blocked energy does to you, firstly at university and more recently with random shooting pains and muscle stress that were classified as Fibromyalgia.

Recover your energy is designed to educate you about what causes fatigue so that you are able to find your own path to wellness. If you are to fully recover and maintain that well-being you need to learn about your own personal energy system. Once you possess that knowledge you can take it with you as you grow into your future. In primary school we learn all about our physical body but nothing really about our emotional and energetic body – this is a sad omission.

All of the *New Perspectives* books have been written for everyone - you don't need any specific knowledge, the book is written as a story from which you will take what you need. You'll certainly find some parts resonate with you more than others and you may find if you re-read it later that sections that didn't hit you on first reading will now "jump off the page" and have a positive effect on you. Learning how to recover your energy will help the wide variety of symptoms you may experience (only some of which are covered in this book) enabling your body to heal itself.

If you need further assistance on any aspect of this work, take a look at the section at the back entitled, **Further Assistance For You And Others**. I am always only too pleased to help your recovery to wellness.

You may also find the web-site helpful www.empoweringhealth.co.uk and you can contact me via email olive@empoweringhealth.co.uk. If at the moment, reading is simply too much for you, you may prefer to listen to a CD which can be purchased on-line. Further information about the project can be found at www.recoveryourenergy.co.uk

Everyone can visualise

The key to using the energy techniques is to simply follow guided imagery. Everyone can visualise, it's a skill we're born with but may not be in the habit of using. Indeed most people simply aren't aware how to utilise it for the release of energy. Whether you label the pictures you see in your head as your imagination or as visualisation, they are a powerful tool, as individual as everything else about you.

As a child, breathlessly taking in a fairy tale, you never stop to query logistics but just relish the story. Visualisation is about giving your imagination free rein, whether you buy in completely or choose to see a story as a metaphor for all the things that are important and appropriate to you. Don't be afraid to play with ideas and change them to suit you. Don't agonise over reality and truth, this is story-land and reality will only get in the way. Just use this is as a model to work with, letting your mind, body and spirit feel the effects.

Try it out for yourself. Sit comfortably and quietly with your feet flat on the floor, your arms and legs uncrossed and your back fairly straight. Imagine a screen in front of you and on it something very familiar. Maybe your children, a favourite football player, your dog, car, garden, front door or maybe just an apple. See the colour, the shape, the size of this image, see how far away it is from you. Now think about it in a little more detail, let it change slowly into a movie and just watch the action. You may even be able to add sounds and feelings. Notice you can change the colours, the size and the distance; these are your pictures after all.

It doesn't matter whether you see the image clearly, holographically, in 3D, as a cartoon, clearly defined or only hazily. It doesn't even matter if you just pretend you're seeing it. Such is the power of our minds, any of these will work for you.

I look forward very much to hearing from you in the future. Your feedback is invaluable as I move forward with my understanding. I will automatically treat such information confidentially or can incorporate it into my work to help others, as you wish.

Olive Hickmott

Chapter 1: Running on empty

I get up in the morning in a fog, where am I? Am I still partly in my dreams?

I've been told to manage my energy, but I'm running on empty, I don't have any energy to manage.

I have crashes, I don't know why or do I? I have tried to unpack the crashes but I am so *in them* I can't find any clarity and anyway it's too tiring to try.

Then there are those learned people who've never had a crash in their lives who want to argue about the exact label for this illness; is it Yuppy Flu, Myalgic Encephalomyelitis (ME), Chronic Fatigue Syndrome (CFS), Seasonal Affective Disorder (SAD), Post Viral something or other or even un-confirmed Glandular Fever.

What on earth does it matter? I am fatigued and running on empty. And yes, I am angry, I've felt like this for years, and nobody seems to know how to help me – I'm on the *too difficult pile*, and it seems I'm expected to just snap out of it. Huh, I'd like to see them try!

Sometimes I feel I have to get worse before anyone will take me seriously. And then there was that *sweet* consultant who looked me straight in the eye at the age of 14 and said *"you have post-viral syndrome, we can't say how long it will last, could be 2 weeks, 2 months, 2 years or 20 years. And there's nothing we can do to help you it just has to take its course. And you are not to go back to school a bit at a time, wait until you are perfectly confident that you can make it through a whole day."*

Well I never did get back to school and that was 20 years ago, so what the hell am I waiting for? I saw a headline recently *IF IT IS TO BE, IT IS UP TO ME.* I watched the words for some time hoping something would happen, then it slowly dawned on me. I had no idea what to do, all my ideas slid out the window years ago.

It's all so frightening. I'm like the electricity supply, one minute I'm OK, the next my fuses have blown and I can barely stand up so what's happened?

I used to be such an energetic person; rushing here, there and everywhere, 101 things to do, helping others, never a dull moment, full of life.

And look at me now – I've completely lost all that fizz; all I can do is think about how best to get through the day, with what little energy I have; it's horrible. Some days I feel OK after a little exertion and then I'm knocked out for the rest of the week. So I never know whether to try and do more or do less.

Lost in thought, suddenly I heard a voice say "I know what's going on"

"Who said that?"

"I am your little green goblin, And I'm here to point out the blindingly obvious. Things in fact you already know but have simply not connected or known how to react to."

Chapter 2: What green goblins do best

So the little green goblin perched at the bottom of my bed with his head on one side and said,

"I'm here to listen."

"Really, for how long?" I replied, having no idea whether a green goblin was really going to understand me.

"For as long as it takes. Oh, and I've been listening in to what you've been thinking, so you don't need to repeat all that anger again"

"How did you do that?"

"Well, that is what green goblins do best, listen to your thoughts and help you make connections. Actually I've been learning all about you ever since I was parachuted in to help. I organised the headline, made sure you saw it and waited for a good moment when I could be all ears!"

Well, if you've been listening in you probably know as much as I do. Not sure there's very much to add. And my energy won't hold out much longer, so could we be quick?"

"Why don't you just summarise?"

"I've been struggling for years. Some times are better than others; I seem to have a very limited tank of energy and need to ration myself every minute of every day. I'm scared of wasting too much too soon because I know I won't be able to replenish it until I've had some sleep. The trouble is though, when I sleep, the fog often comes back, which makes everything even more difficult.

When the fog's there, I'm completely unable to think. If someone talks to me the words fly past my ears too fast for me to catch. If I try to read, I can't even assemble the words in my head to make a sentence.

Then there's the pain that randomly arrives in any part of my body, sometimes like moving pins and needles, and at other times almost like a series of electric shocks. I have no idea what any of this is all about. On a couple of occasions I have had continuous pain for days. Some people have said it's fibromyalgia, but another label probably won't help, so I just put up with it. And now my mother who has been popping in to look after me for years isn't well, so she needs my energy too, but I honestly haven't got enough for both of us.

Also I seem to be suffering from more and more allergic reactions and food intolerances. I have to cut out so many foods I just can't enjoy a meal any more. I don't know what on earth I can eat without worrying. And then mum keeps on at me for not eating enough, saying that's why I lack energy. So I've been eating goodness knows what and of course have put on weight which I think makes me even more tired. Whatever I eat seems to go straight to fat. Food doesn't seem to give me any energy at all, more often the reverse. So I'm totally baffled as to what to do.

When I last saw my local doctor, I felt he was tolerating me thinking 'Another sad woman - hysterical nonsense'. Of course that only made me more angry and confused.

Sometimes I wonder if I really have the right to be on the planet at all. I think there might be something in me that's saying "*You don't deserve any energy*", maybe this is a payoff for bad behaviour when I was a kid. At this point it all gets too scary and I try to block it out but that in itself takes so much effort. "

"Could you take a deep breath?" asked the goblin, "It will help you to naturally slow down a little? Breathing is actually rather good for you!"

"Actually." I admitted, "I probably often stop breathing, especially when things are getting more and more confused in my mind. Mind you, getting all this out of my system helps. It's as if I can see all my problems over there on the table, which is where I'd like it to be – right away from me. Can a green goblin really help?"

The goblin nodded his head, "I can certainly help you understand what's going on and how you can move forward. What do you think your life would be like if you were better?"

"That's a difficult one. I fell ill as a teenager, never got any GCSEs etc and have no job. Who would I be if I were well? Scary thought to cope with."

"Well," said the goblin, "Gwendolyn, the good fairy will be popping along to help you with that side of things. I'm your own personal goblin; my job's to help you recognise what's really going on. You see, part of you wants to get out of bed, but part of you yearns to stay. Part of you wants to go ahead with your life, part of you just wants to pull the duvet over your head and give up. There are so many parts of you in conflict with each other. *The Team* is trained to tackle all this confusion."

"Sorry? *The Team?*"

"Certainly. Your *Support Team*. You'll be meeting them, one at a time over the next few days. Not to worry, they're all really cool and total experts when it comes to you. But I must get on with my own job. What do you think causes your energy crashes?"

"No idea."

"Can you recall one of your crashes, which is just a symptom, and trace it backwards to find the cause, go back as far as you need, perhaps 5 minutes, maybe 5 hours."

"Well, very often I'll get a visitor who comes to see me, tells me how awful I look and then they'll dump a load of their misery on me and as if that wasn't bad enough they'll then tell me all about everyone else they know who's really tired too. By the time they've gone I feel dreadful. But I can't tell them not to come, or I wouldn't get any visitors at all."

"So you're left holding all their negative energy?"

"What are my options? I can't cut myself off from everyone."

"That's not what I'm suggesting." The goblin leaned forward, head on his hand, concentrating. "How long does it take for you to crash? What sets it off? Can it be brought on by listening to music, watching the soaps or worse still the news?"

"Well funny you should mention that, there certainly seem to be more than the usual load of disasters lately. I was thinking perhaps I just shouldn't watch them because sometimes I feel physically sick."

"And then?"

"Then I end up in bed for hours. But not knowing what's going on in the outside world makes me feel as if I'm becoming a recluse."

"What's your reaction to a disaster-ridden news programme?"

"Miserable, sad, frustrated I'm helpless to do anything. I'm often angry."

"So, you get a load of other people's misery and at other times you're getting bad energy from your own reactions to outside events.

Added to that you're trying to take all their troubles onto your own shoulders. Quite a load?"

" That's just who I am I suppose. When anyone in the family's unhappy, I feel dreadful. I so much want to be able to sort them out but I haven't even got enough energy to set myself straight. And then I crash, all energy vanishes and I don't know what to do except sleep it off; it's like all my fuses are blown.

The Goblin nodded his understanding, paused a moment then said "Can you think of your energy distributed all over your body like the fairy lights on a Christmas tree? You have hundreds of lights or meridian points, and just like annoying Christmas tree lights, if one goes out it's likely the next few will go too.

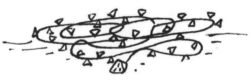

To get your energy flowing, you need to have all your lights on, clearing blockages. Your energy gets blocked through operations, accidents, emotions, stress, other people's energy (when they dump on us), It can be blocked by negative life experiences and limiting beliefs, The most popular personal energy model has at least 7 main junction boxes, just like the main fuse box in your home. These are called chakras.[2] The negative energy builds up in your cells, causing a decreasing energy

---

[2] You will see a note on page 353 of *You Too Can 'Do' Health!* explaining where they are located in western traditions.

until your chakras get really blocked; then we see time and time again patterns of illness and disease forming."[3]

"So you're saying that either I pick up other people's negative energy or I generate my own? And that's what blows my fuses? Do you know that's exactly what it feels like, as if the mains connector has been unplugged."

"And what about physical exercise? Do you manage any?"

"Not really. I've been told to conserve the energy I have and ration myself. They call that *fatigue management*. It's second nature now after all these years."

"If you're running on empty anyway, physical exercise is only going to tip you over the top. But wouldn't it be so much better if you were practising *energy management*, isn't that a far more positive approach? The term *fatigue management* makes you feel exhausted from the start because you're internally re-enforcing that *fatigue* message."

"The mornings are so hard, I'm like a zombie - I've discovered this word that describes it perfectly — DISCOMBOBULATED. Most days it takes until lunchtime before I've come round. I read this book on dreams and sleep levels and feel I never get to the important level 4 when your body has an opportunity to repair itself. I feel as if I've spent the whole night busily dreaming, I can't remember details but I know they're not happy dreams. When I wake up I feel more fatigued than I did when I went to sleep."

The Goblin nodded his head again,

---

[3] *You too can 'do' health!*

"If you've read about sleep and dreams you'll know dreams often focus on unresolved issues in your life. Repetitive dreams are issues popping up again and again because they aren't being addressed. It may be that you don't want to face the problems or that at some level you feel they are insoluble. Dreams are dealt with by the right side of the brain and can easily be forgotten in the first few minutes of awakening. So you need a pen and paper beside your bed to make a note. I know when you wake up you're in a bit of a fog but Maisey will be really impressed if you write some of your dreams down. They could be very useful"

"Who on earth is Maisey?" I asked.

"Oh, she's the daughter of that internationally renowned detective (can't mention his name) who's always solving clues and tracking down villains. Maisey's followed in her father's footsteps, except she concentrates on tracking down clues that are inside you. Once you've found the patterns causing your ill health, everything starts to make sense and you can make changes to find real wellness."

"Where do I find her?"

"Don't worry. She'll appear when you're ready. And while we're on the subject of your right brain, what metaphors do you use to describe yourself?"

"Sorry?"

"Pet phrases you use?"

"I'm sick and tired of being ill. That the sort of thing you mean?"

"Certainly is. And when were you first sick and tired?"

"Well, I remember feeling that way about my new school, before I even started!"

"So you became sick and tired quite literally."

"Hadn't really thought about it like that."

"Well you should. People often keep giving themselves a message and eventually their body believes it and they physically manifest exactly what they've been thinking about.

I remember one chap I helped. He used to tell himself he was sick to the stomach of an ongoing situation in his life. One day he developed a tremendous pain in his abdomen. He thought he had appendicitis. The interesting thing was that while he was manifesting being *sick to the stomach* all his negative emotions left him. The pain raged until he got home. Then it went and the negative emotions returned. You see, manifesting a thought can override strong emotion. Can you recall any other descriptive words you tend to use about yourself?"

I gave it some thought,

"I often say how drained I am and how I have no energy."

"Ah, common triggers for fatigue. Watch out! You have to learn how to get rid of those or they will continually hold you back. Have you ever had a time when you felt really well?"

" Mum and Dad took me on holiday once. I didn't think I'd even make it up the stairs to the plane. We went to the Maldives, in the Indian Ocean. As I got off the plane, in glorious sunshine, I seemed to have left all the bad feelings and fatigue behind. We had a great two weeks, sunshine, scenery, lovely food and super people. But in the car from the airport home I could feel it all coming back. I'd forgotten about that."

"It's important to keep an experience like that alive, so your mind has the opportunity even now to compare and contrast what it was that made such a difference to you. Whoops!"

The Goblin suddenly leapt up from his position at the bottom of my bed, making me jump.

"Time I made myself scarce, Edward, the personal energy repair electrician is heading this way. He has so much energy, little people like me sometimes start fizzing around the ceiling."

And suddenly, the little green goblin whirled round once, waved and flew out of the window.

Chapter 3: Edward the electrician

Before I could even think why there should be an electrician in the house, the door flew open and in bounced a rather rounded chap bearing a big gold toolbox and a bigger smile.

"Hello Hello, Edward's the name, electrical problems the game. Come to help you fix your connections. I see you don't have any energy, probably running on empty. How much of the energy running your body is your's right now?"

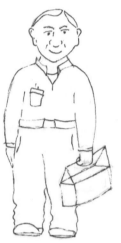

Before I could think, the number 20% popped up in my mind. I could actually see a dial with a lever marked at the 20% level.

"Actually I think that may be a wee bit optimistic, but no matter." said Edward.

"Just make sure the 20% is your energy right now, not energy from some time in the past."

"Gosh, 10% just popped up then, but that sounds really dreadful!"

"Not to worry, not to worry! We can fix it. It's just always helpful to have an idea of exactly where you are before you try to get where you want to be. "

"But where are these numbers coming from?"

"Oh, straight from your subconscious, and you should congratulate yourself for doing such a great job of telling yourself what's going on. When you pick up negative energy from others, it will always be their energy and you can't possibly run your body on energy that belongs to other people and particularly if it's the wrong sort - it just makes you feel odd and blows your fuses.

Of course, if you have something that's worrying you – could have happened last week, last year or even years ago - that event could be leaking negative energy from inside. Think about it, anything like that lying around? Whether it's twenty years old or a few weeks old, it's *too* old, it's draining, past its sell-by, and you're going to be much better off without it."

"What about that dreadful doctor? I'm still angry with him more than 20 years later!"

"And that's helping you how? What good's it doing? Does he care? I don't think so! Does he even remember? What do you think? So why waste time on him? Let go and just hope he's grown a little wiser as he got older. "

"Easier said than done." I could hear how grumpy I sounded.

"Now, now, try not to be judgemental. Probably said what he did with the best of intentions. If you can just see he was only trying to help, you'll find it easier to let go. And don't worry, I have some great tools that will help you shift some of the stale stuff and you can have fun at the same time. Ready? Well, here we go, just slowly to start with.

Think of your energy as a river, a natural flow of energy.

Always make sure your arms and legs are uncrossed to get the best flow.

If the flow isn't strong enough, rubbish builds up.

If the blocks are large enough, the river is forced to re-route - I can teach you to release those blocks and manage both the inflow and outflow of your energy. If the outflow is blocked the inflow will stop too. It's natural self regulation.

In times of flood, water may be lost and never find its way back to the river - I can teach you to recover your energy from places it's trickled away to. I'm going to give you all the tools you need to maintain energy. You wouldn't dream of not brushing your teeth and washing every day, shouldn't you be cleaning your energy field too? Just because most people can't see it, you can still sense it and know when it needs a good going-over. You can't see gravity or the wind but you can certainly feel them, they're just different forms of energy."

"So have I got a lot of rubbish blocking my energy flow?"

"A lorry-load! Let's see if this helps."

With a huge whoosh, a large golden cloud burst out of the gold toolbox and started dancing around the room.

It was like watching a magic spring clean in action; it finally settled in the 8 corners of the room, floor and ceiling, ran little threads to meet in the centre, paused a moment and then dived down through the floor deep into the ground and right down to the centre of the earth, leaving the room sparkling with a great feeling of peace.

"Is that what you do?" I asked in amazement.

"Just a starter!" Edward did his best but failed to look in the least bit modest, "Now you."

"Me?"

"Just think about it happening. Energy follows thought. Imagine pulling in gold energy and imagine it doing what you've just seen. You can do it your own way if you like, energy loves creativity."

I concentrated hard,

"This is incredible ..." speechless, I watched the torrent of golden energy clean the room, shoot from one corner to another, assemble in the middle and dive into the earth.

"Wow! Did I do that?"

"Everyone can, just needs a little imagination. I can guide you through all sorts of things to imagine and you can have lots of fun using them yourself. How are you feeling now?"

"Not much different in terms of energy but I certainly feel calmer, less frantic in my head. Also I had a rather odd feeling of dropping into the bed."

"That's you feeling more connected to your body, grounded rather than being up in your head with hundreds of thoughts running around. As you progress you'll find that connection getting stronger and you'll feel calmer, more focused."

"That's very reassuring, so why was the green goblin so nervous of you?"

"Oh, he used to love to join the gold energy running around the room, but one person we met zapped it so fast the first time that he got knocked out. So I always ask people to run it gently, because it's a very powerful concept. You can always increase the flow later. The goblin is still a bit wary of people trying it for the first time. As you learn to direct your energy it's important you don't impose it on others.

Now let's start to release and eliminate some of that old energy that's hanging around from other people. As we progress you'll be releasing lots of energy and I certainly don't want to take all that away with me. We're going to use the concept of a magnet in a ring of fire that can simply burn up all this unwanted energy."

Just imagine a huge magnet, make it whatever colour or shape you like, making sure it's good and strong. Surround it with a ring of fire and pass the magnet down your front, say about 2/3 feet from your body. Just let the magnet attract any old emotions, negative energy, old programming, karma, food intolerances, phobias, limiting beliefs... All the stuff that you no longer need; that's right -just watch it go, hear it go or feel it go, any of these will be just perfect. [4]

Now, if you feel anything blocking you doing this, just let go of the block.

---

[4] In the New Perspectives book, *You too can 'do' health!,* page 173, there is some guided imagery with a lake and a magnet. That is another alternative if you prefer.

If nothing is happening, just release the block that is blocking the block.

If you still don't feel that anything's working, release the block that's blocking the block, that's blocking the block!

By this time there will be nothing left to block anything.

You don't control it, it will all happen, just as it does when you sit in a cinema or theatre. You have no control over the film or play, you're just experiencing it. This experience could be in the form of pictures, cartoon images, sounds or feelings, whatever appeals to your subconscious.

You won't need to worry that you'll be losing something you still need, your subconscious is very conservative and it won't let you release anything that you might regret losing. It's far more likely to keep things you don't need than lose anything you do.

Now just let the magnet do its work attracting old emotions, negative energy and old programming out of the front of your body, and let the fire just burn these up. Now let the magnet travel down the back of you, where lots of "clutter" often hides, attracting and burning up old emotions, negative energy, limiting beliefs, karma and old programming. Continue down your right side, your left side, above your head and below your feet. Now, how was that?"

"Really odd. I saw lots of **stuff** rushing away from me and burning up."

"And how do you feel now?"

"OK! And I've just read my meter and I now have 25% of my own energy running my body...this is simply amazing: how did that happen?"

"Simply cleaning your energy field. I can see it's a lot clearer than it was, and there's more to do yet. 25% may be a little optimistic when you realise exactly what is really your energy. Don't worry; it will adjust as you practice more.

Would you be able to do that same process twice a day, once when you get up and once before going to sleep? It will really make a difference. Any time you feel *lit up* by strong emotions it's really good to straightaway put out a new magnet, clear it and fill up the gap with more new golden energy."

"Just a minute. When you were talking earlier, I was beginning to feel really tired, but that seems to be getting better now. I feel I can keep chatting for a bit longer. This is really easy."

"Now it's time to start recovering your energy, from wherever you have scattered it. Some people get told by their family and friends that the only solution is to pull themselves together and you will be alright."

"Don't say that! That's exactly the sort of thing that really annoys me!"

"Hang on a minute; let's think about what I actually said. The thought of pulling yourself together in itself is a fascinating concept. If you and your energy are not together, where are you? People also use the expression *feeling all over the place,* so where have they left parts of themselves?

If you're worrying about your mother, are you leaving your energy with her, or with other people you know?"

"Oh yes, I've always felt that I should give my mum and others all the energy they want from me, that's why I used to be so manic. I thought I was generating more."

"Being manic keeps you in your head and not grounded; a very stressful feeling and it may stop energy flowing in through your feet into your main energy channels. First things first. Let's see about recovering your energy."

"Oh no, I can't do that, my mum needs it! I'd feel very guilty just taking it away, with no warning."

"No problem."

I was just picturing my mum standing there without my energy. She was looking very sad and a bit deflated. But at that moment Edward pressed another button on his toolbox. Suddenly there was a gold ball of shining energy above her head, sparkling and dancing. As I watched, it slowly cascaded down over and into her body and she was smiling. I also saw with surprise, my own energy flowing back to me.

"You see, once you introduced her to Universal Gold energy, she liked it a lot and was happy to give yours back. It's important you just offer it to her to take if she wants. If she doesn't want the Universal Gold energy, then assure her it will just evaporate in a couple of days."

"But I didn't do anything."

"Oh yes you did. All you had to do was to think about the energy and there it was. ENERGY FOLLOWS THOUGHT.

Now before you accept that energy back into you, imagine a gold ball of energy above your head, let it collect any energy that you've scattered with anyone, left in distant places etc., clean it up, make it really sparkling and let it just beam back onto the top of your head and fill up all the gaps that have been left when you released all that negative stuff.[5] How do you feel now?"

"Wow, now I have about 40% of my own energy and I feel a whole lot better."

"Great! And I think that's enough for today. Collect in your energy field to about 3 to 5 feet around you, just like a lovely soft duvet. That will keep you safe and start to protect you from other energies. Practise what you have been learning and I'll see you again when you've done some detective work with Maisey. Now I'm going to take the scenic route."

So saying, he disappeared inside his toolbox which rose and glided like a golden spaceship right out of the window.

I must have dozed off then into a really relaxed and comfortable sleep, until I woke up bright and alert. I could hear a little voice calling,

"Cooee! Cooee ! It's Maisey here!"...

---

[5] The full version of all of these guided imageries is available on a CD, that can be purchased from www.empoweringhealth.co.uk.

Chapter 4: Maisey investigates

Maisey sat down. She was a petite woman, trim and neat, her clothes obviously carefully chosen. There was an air of effortless efficiency about her.

"I have to channel your curiosity," she began.

"Oh but I've done that, thought all round the problem - Why do I deserve this? What have I done? Why me? on and on till my head spins. I've thought so much I even wonder if I've made up things that aren't really true."

Maisey held up her hand,

"Hang on! This is all very interesting but none of this is about blame! None at all! It's about investigation. We don't need to blame anything or anyone. That's a waste of time, effort and especially energy. What we need are the facts of the case. Tell me what was going on in your life just before you started to feel ill?"

"I was really busy. I was rushed off my feet, always playing sport, the family had just moved house, about 100 miles, and I had gone to a new school."

"Aha! There goes another metaphor. Being rushed off your feet – sounds very ungrounded. Edward will help you to ground and let go of that metaphor later. And what time of year was this? "

"We had moved in late July, gone on holiday in August and I had started a new school in September."

"Were you looking forward to the new school?"

"Yes and no. I was going to be in the same school as my brother and that was good, but at the same time a bit scary. I wouldn't know anyone, he's a lot older, I had to go on the school bus and when I went for a trial day I got completely lost. "

"How did getting lost make you feel?"

"Terrified! I was sure I'd never see my family again. Finally a nice teacher reunited me with the girl who should have been looking after me. Thinking about it now I wonder if my memory has made it even scarier than it was."

"Before we go any further let me tell you a little trick for your memory. We really don't know the difference between fact and fiction. If for example you dream your car had been stolen you would look out the window and check. Well if you make up a picture in your memory make sure you always sign it, then you will know whether you have made it up. Try it out for a moment with your imagination and see if it works for you."

"This is really fun, I feel like an artist and all my own pictures have a lovely signature."

"Now going back to that nasty experience in school, you need to realise it's not the experience in itself that's the most important thing, but your reaction to it. This reaction, and the importance you give it caused you stress whenever you thought about it, whether consciously or unconsciously. All that stress, on its own, can make you completely fatigued."

"You are right. I 'm feeling tired just thinking about that dreadful day. I honestly don't think I can talk much longer. "

"That's great! "

"What! It's not great at all! What on earth's great about it?"

"Great opportunity to clear some negative energy. Get out one of those huge magnets. You've just *lit up* a whole lot of energy. Now sit back and just let it all clear."

As I sat back against the pillows, running the guided imagery, this time I imagined a magnet in a deep lake. I saw lots of books, school books going off to the magnet. Then there was other stuff leaving - I couldn't see it but I could feel it leaving. Then I felt a pain in my neck as something got stuck, so I asked to release the block and it went immediately. I'd always thought that moving to a new school was a pain in the neck! I noticed I was feeling lighter and my neck was more flexible.

"You're doing really well. Still want to stop?"

"No, I'd really like to finish my story now. I'd had a really lovely holiday and the minute I got back I was really ill. I suppose it was a tummy bug I'd picked up. I was so tired I had to stay in bed for 4 days. When I got up I just seemed to have lost all my sparkle.

I dragged myself around for the next few weeks and eventually, one day at school I became so tired, I just knew I couldn't hack it any more. For a few months I tried really hard to keep going, I was off school and by the time I eventually met that consultant, I went home and all I could do was to sit and cry. It felt just like a death sentence.

I was only 14. I had no prospect of health and happiness and eventually I didn't even have enough energy to cry."

"Just a moment- now, just start releasing some more of this negative emotion that's having such an effect on you. You know how to do it and this is a great opportunity to get it out of your body, out of your cells. You are really *lit up* now. Whenever you feel an emotion, you have the option to suppress it, express it (normally by getting angry or upset), or release it. Releasing it is the way to go if you want to be healthy - That's right, let it all go, as much as is now prepared to leave. Just send it all to the magnet."

I could feel loads and loads of stuff just pouring off me – through my whole body - my chest, my abdomen, my legs and feet. I was wondering when it would ever stop.

Then I noticed a gold ball of positive healing energy hovering above my head, generating some lovely gold and turquoise sparkly energy and it was gently falling onto my head. As it ran through my body I felt a gorgeous warm glow coursing through my veins, filling up all the gaps.

"Wow! That was totally amazing!"

"You see, whenever negative energy *lights up* for you, that's a great opportunity to release it; it has just bubbled up to the surface. Instead of being drained by it, take it as a present, an opportunity to do some good housekeeping of your energy system."

I gulped hard, it wasn't necessarily my idea of a present but I knew it needed to be done.

"So, to summarise, you had a big change in your life, giving you quite a bit of stress, and maybe that holiday virus was just *the last straw.*"

"Well, now you say it like that it all seems very simple. But all that happened years ago! What keeps me in this stuck state? Surely my immune system should have got me out of it by now?"

"Well that depends."

"On what?"

"A lot of things; we all get ill from time to time, but the secret of wellness is recovery."

"And I *should* be able to hack this, shouldn't I?"

"Give yourself a break for a minute. The word *should* is just signalling to yourself that you're a failure. That sort of talk won't help at all!"

"Just a minute! I'm always doing it! I tell myself I *should* get up, I *should* go out, I *should* wash my hair today..."

"And what do you feel like when you issue these commands? Try one now."

"You're right! I feel ghastly! I'd better release some more to the magnet."

This time I could just see puffs of smoke disappearing into the lake.

"How do you feel now?"

"Tired, but a different sort of tired. I think I need a nap. This seems to be a comfortable tired feeling. I feel very relaxed."

"Great! You've started to really understand what's been happening and you're already taking steps to change things."

"Zzzzzzzzz...!"

Chapter 5: Maisey re-educates the Captain

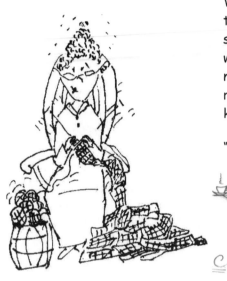

When I awoke, Maisey was still there. She was knitting. It was something very brightly coloured. I was listening to the click of the needles. It's a very soothing rhythm when someone is good at knitting.

"I don't mean to be rude, but why are you still here and what are you knitting? "

"Oh, you mentioned your immune system and I thought we should do a little investigation on that too. I just love knitting, it's very relaxing, much better than watching TV, and I can use this scarf to demonstrate something very important to you about your immune system."

That made no sense to me at all, but by this time nothing really did and I hoped everything would become clear.

"Now you mentioned your immune system *should* have got you out of it by now. Can you explain a little more?"

"Well, it's clearly useless at its job. Whoops! There's another belief!"

"What else?"

"Well it should have helped me get over a virus and it's proved useless. It's as if it's been on holiday for the last 20 years."

"What do you know about your immune system?"

"Not a lot, maybe I haven't even got one!"

"Well, your immune system is a learning organisation. It learns every moment of every day. For example, when you had chicken pox it learnt about that and put the information in a metaphorical filing cabinet so whenever you came in contact again with that virus, all the correct fighting information poured out of the cabinet in your defence. So you never got it again.

"So do we conclude my stupid immune system has gone on strike - hasn't learnt anything for 20 years?"

Maisey frowned

"Imagine you were talking to a child who was having difficulty learning something – is that the sort of thing you'd say to them?"

"Oh no, of course not, that would be a dreadful thing to do,"

"But it's OK to tell yourself something like that?"

"No, I suppose not but I always give myself a hard time. Perhaps I'd try to explain things in a different way, so the child could understand and get it right next time. I 'd never call them stupid. Anyway, they're just having a struggle with something. That doesn't make them stupid."

"OK, so how could you explain to your immune system how to get it right? "

I must have looked completely dumbfounded and there was a bit of a pause, while I racked my brains to try and shine some light on the challenge of talking to my immune system.

"Well, I might try to give a child a small step first. I guess communicating in pictures might be an idea. Most things seem to work best in pictures."

"Excellent. And what would be a suitable picture for how your immune system feels right now?"

"A shipwreck. There is a little bit functioning in complete isolation, with a flashing distress light on the top, going around in circles. Everything else is just bits of wood, floating about in the sea. Lots of rubbish lying around and no direction at all."

"And how would you like it to be?"

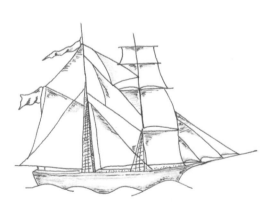

"A beautiful old fashioned sailing boat, drifting majestically across the ocean; just going with the ebb and flow of the waves and currents." But when I think of that happening, **Impossible** is the word that springs to mind."

"How would you teach a

child? Your immune system is a fast learner once it gets clear instruction and realises the current state is not ideal. And look, I've dropped a stitch in the scarf, it'll keep laddering down to the bottom if I don't teach it how to repair itself, stitch by stitch and get back onto the needles."

"Actually Maisey, that makes it really clear now. A step by step approach to wellness, just like picking up one stitch at a time. And as you said before, when you were telling me how everyone gets ill at some time or other, it's really a question of how they go about becoming well again.

I suppose I could suggest that the boat first finds all the floating odds and ends. Maybe just start with finding the large ones, a bit like a jigsaw puzzle, and then pull in the others to fit. I would need to check that all the bits really belonged to my boat and they weren't just driftwood, because that would make the re-build very confusing. Hey, that reminds me of what Edward was saying to me about pulling myself together.

Having found all the bits it needs much stronger glue, nails and reinforcing. Where do I get these?"

"Just set the intent that you can find the strong stuff you need to make it whole in your imagination and see what happens."

"It really is pulling itself together, just like a jigsaw, and everything is being bound into place. It looks, sounds and feels a lot stronger now. And now there's a pile of old stuff in the tug that no longer fits the boat, maybe from before the last refit or maybe from another boat. Either way it's no longer needed and can be taken away for recycling."

"Now it needs a good clean out. Let's use some of Edward's gold energy and run it around every nook and cranny in the boat, sparkling it up. The rubbish is just being thrown overboard into that waiting tug.

"So it's gathered together, it has deleted all the stuff that doesn't belong, it's stronger and it's cleaner. What next?"

"It needs fitting out with new equipment and a crew to run it – all the old ones deserted years ago."

"Just take a survey around the boat and order up and install all the resources you want; it's your boat."

"Excellent! This is like a fabulous shopping spree and no budget restrictions. And I need a new crew, who've been properly trained, to update the original blueprints for the boat with up to date information.

The training won't be immediate but I can hear the Project Manager saying it will be a careful process, with incremental changes over the next month and then HMS Immune will be fully functional. Is that really all I need to do?"

"You've done a great job. One last thing. It's important to make sure that captain and crew are all aligned with the same priorities and goal; you want to minimise any conflict[6], room for indecision and confusion. Like with any other programme where a lot of change is involved, remember you are the captain of the ship and you may need to remind the team of some of the principles, leave them to the details, and check how they're getting on, from time to time, perhaps daily to start with."

---

[6] A practitioner can easily assist you to resolve any major internal conflicts.

"Wait a minute, I can see some signs with **INTOLERANCE** written on them, being thrown into a waiting tug that is collecting the rubbish. What does that mean? "

"Often people who have a compromised immune system develop intolerances to food, airborne smells, chemicals etc. It's normally due to real confusion in your immune system and it's trying to cope the best it can. Over the next month you may find your food intolerances reduce as your immune system picks up. That work you did on cleaning with Edward will be working too. You will know when it is time to start slowly re-introducing them"

"Sometimes I feel quite intolerant about several things, not only food intolerances."

"I wasn't going to mention those yet but since it's come up do you think there's a connection? Are you manifesting food intolerance from emotional intolerance? It can happen."

"Well that is going to really change things!"

"How does your immune system feel now?"

"Much stronger and more knowledgeable, and I can see lots of work going on in the boat."

"Can you imagine when it is sailing across the sea and using its new strength to take it through the waves, wind, rain, sunshine etc without being knocked off course – in fact, all the ups and downs of modern living. Boats are safe in harbour, but that is not where they're designed to stay."

"Now don't forget to give yourself a new lake and magnet and let go of anything that has *lit up*, I can see there is some ready to go now. Gather up your energy, especially out of my space and any that you have left elsewhere, shine it up, bring in some new golden energy and let it shine back into your body through the top of your head."

With that I relaxed into the chair in what felt like perfect peace. I was really starting to appreciate how these guided meditations were relaxing and renewing me.

Later I really wanted to tidy up a bit, so I pottered around but there was still this nagging voice in my head asking whether this was really a good idea. After watching the TV for a little I eventually gave in and went to bed.

Chapter 6: Edward re-connects the mains

It must have been about 12 noon the next day before I awoke. Maybe I *came around* a little bit quicker than normal but I seemed to have gone backwards a little from yesterday. The pains in my body, the constant reminder, were there again, just as usual. I hobbled into the living room and collapsed in the armchair.

I saw a gold ball on the mantelpiece and remembered Edward's words "Do this twice a day." Well I haven't got anything to lose, I thought, so I straightened myself up, created a lake to put the magnet in and sat back.

I wasn't awake enough yet to direct my thoughts; it was like watching a movie. The lake appeared amongst snow capped mountains, the slopes covered in fir trees, little cartoon characters were marching along the track, singing, "Hi ho!, hi ho! It's off to work we go!" and jumping, one at a time, into the lake. It was like a scene I had never seen from Snow White.

They were really happy and were bouncing into the lake as if released from a spring board. I found myself giggling and remembered Edward saying "The more fun you can have with your pictures the better."

There were a lot more than 7 dwarfs, nearer 700 I would think. They were all marching happily behind one another in a long line. Eventually the column came to an end with really tiny characters. I was distracted just watching the cartoons, when I felt that familiar whoosh come into the room. It was Edward riding his gold toolbox. He tossed a large gold ball into the air, mixed it with lots of purple and lilac and it fell dreamily onto my head and down into my body.

"You must always remember to re-fill with energy or you leave a vacuum and nature abhors a vacuum. You certainly don't want all that stuff you've just released to come back, so it's quite simple to fill up with some really positive energy. Gold is the simplest but if you look above the gold you may notice a brilliant circular rainbow. Pick any colour you like from to add to your gold energy so it becomes exactly the kind of energy you're seeking at this moment. "So how are you now?"

"A lot better since some more stuff just left. Is there any limit to the amount of stuff that needs to go? Am I really clearing the system or just making more?"

"You've had a lot of clogged energy, you know that, and you've got a lot of *cupboards* to clear. Maybe nobody ever lets go of 100%, and you will collect more, but at the moment you're doing a full spring clean and it will take time. However we're talking days and weeks, not months and years. Today I just want to make sure you can get your feet on the floor"

"Of course I can get my feet on the floor, how do you think I got to this armchair?"

"Well, I notice you now have your feet on a footstool, and I need to help you connect with the earth's energy as well as universal energy."

"Hang on a minute, how many energies are there?"

"All the obvious ones like gravity, sunshine and the wind. You can't see any of them although you can feel the sun and wind. Energy such as gravity you take for granted although if it didn't work we'd certainly notice that.

Some people can actually see, in their mind's eye, energies that others just don't notice. For example, Faraday, the inventor, could actually see lines of electromagnetic force[7]. I can see your energy and it's looking better already. But it doesn't seem to be very active through your legs. Tell me about the pain you get."

"I often get shooting pains that stop as suddenly as they start. And you can't tell the doctor about them as they move about and they're rarely in the same place, so he'd just say it's my imagination."

"It's not your imagination, it's energy blocks, and I'm going to help you clear these right now. Firstly, I need you to put your feet on the ground."

"OK that's not difficult"

"Just notice if you have any strong emotions; connect with yourself for a moment, what do you feel like?"

"I'm getting a bit irritated."

"Any idea why?"

"No, but now I'm feeling frustrated as well."

"That'll be because you've put your legs on the ground. This often happens with blocked energy, especially in those with Chronic Fatigue for some reason."

He pressed the eject button on his gold toolbox and a bronze star appeared in the middle of the room.

---

[7] *The mind's eye*, Page 31

"Just imagine you can put all that irritation, frustration and anything else that is connected into the star, and send it off to the other side of the moon."

"It's gone! And the emotion has gone too!" What happened there?

Edward smiled,

"You just released the energy around a specific emotion. You can use it for beliefs too."

"Extraordinary! And could I get rid of that belief about my energy being rationed?"

"Just think about the belief, imagine it as some object, any object will do. If nothing comes to mind just use a rose, and then destroy the rose, send it to the other side of the moon, blow it up, whatever works for you. That's a very quick way to lose beliefs you don't want and are no longer appropriate.

In exactly the same way you can destroy some of those old metaphors and beliefs about *being drained, not deserving your energy* etc as a little homework whenever you want to.

Now fill up with new sparking gold energy from above, so you don't have a vacuum. How are your legs feeling now they're on the ground?"

"Not great, but I'll hang on in there, clear everything else that pops up and see what happens next."

"I want to reconnect your whole energy system by teaching you to run your energy through your body, clearing any blocks you find. This will be universal energy from above and also the earth's energy from below you.

Just imagine a seed germinating in the soil for a moment. First it grows little roots down into the soil, and there is an exchange - nutrition comes up into the seed and waste products return to the earth. Then it starts to sprout above the soil fed by energy from above and in particular sunlight. So there we have a perfect metaphor of how our energy system needs to connect to earth and universal energy.

OK, let's give it a go. Firstly I should like to explain to you a bit more about grounding."

"Is that why people say keep your feet on the ground?"

"Yes, being grounded helps us to live in the present, rather than worrying about the past or what might be in the future. We can just enjoy what's going on around us in the here and now."

It is about keeping feet on the ground, feeling connected to your body, aware of your body and moving that chaotic action out of your head and into the calmer waters of your body"

At that very moment and with a huge rumbling a large tree crashed into the room, standing upright as if it were meant to be there.

"Just take a look at the roots of this tree; they go right down into the ground."

And sure enough, it was as if I had X-ray eyes! I could see them going further and further down into the ground, searching out the centre of the earth.

"A tree gets nourishment from the earth and passes waste materials back into the earth.

Just like a tree, imagine you have roots that reach down into the centre of the earth. Feel your body slightly sink as you become firmly attached to the ground, to the centre of the earth and spread them out to make the tree really firm. As you do this you will feel nurturing energy coming up through your feet and at the same time you're giving negative emotions, programming, limiting beliefs, etc...the opportunity to sink down into the ground."

"This is great! I feel much more connected to the ground now."

"Take a drink of water that will help you to feel grounded. You can even imagine catching all those busy thoughts in your hand and moving them down your belly."

Getting up and walking about I really did feel **more grounded**, then I walked over to hug the tree and became even more firmly attached.

"You're using the tree's roots. You can get that level of stability just through your own imagination. Your own inner wisdom will know the perfect way to ground you. Just think of a gymnast they are very aware of where their body is, even if they are tumbling and when they land they become firmly connected to the ground in an instant. Some people take a walk in the forest or even just imagine doing that and immediately feel grounded.

So now your energy system is grounded, firmly connected to the earth and you can feel present. Even the domestic electricity is grounded to provide a stable energy system."

"And the more I ground, the less busy my brain feels. I have sort of sunk down about an inch and my whole body feels more relaxed, my muscles are no longer in tension. Magic!"

At that moment a few more emotions popped up, so I put them in the star and dispatched them to the other side of the moon.

"Nice one, you really are getting this. That feeling of being able to relax your muscles will help the muscle pain. Being too much in your head and not enough in your body is a very stressful place, both physically and mentally. Please take a seat again. Now you are grounded, I can teach you about universal and ground energy – you needed to ground first.

So just take a couple of easy deep breaths, relax your jaw muscles, relax the point on your forehead between your eyebrows, relax your chest, relax your pelvic area, relax your knees and relax your feet."

At these words, I did my best to follow Edward's instructions. I wondered vaguely whether I was about to blow up with all the effort, but before I could follow this thought, I heard Edward saying, "Just relax, this is a space of no effort and miracles." Then he pressed a button with a picture of a person on it.

On the wall in front of me I saw myself, sitting on a chair, back straight, arms and legs uncrossed on the surface of a huge holographic picture of the world. From the centre of the earth, full of giant hot crystals and molten bubbling rocks was a bright light beaming up into the soles of my feet. It was swirling around entering my feet through little holes in my heels, my insteps and my toes. It was quite exciting to just watch what would happen next, just like watching a movie unfurl before my eyes and I didn't have to do anything. The energy passed into my feet, ankles and calves, and as it travelled along Edward said,

"It will be cleaning and clearing your energy centres and energy channels of limiting beliefs, old pictures, old programming, negative events, old karma – everything you no longer need that is not your energy, and not in the present time – TODAY.

I watched the picture evolve, like a photograph developing. More and more energy was coming in and swirling through my limbs, through my knees, thighs, pelvis, up the front of my body all the way to my ribs and then down my back to my pelvis again, where it collected into a ball of energy. I heard Edward saying,

"Now, imagine the centre of the earth reaching up to the base of your spine with its force of gravity, and allow it to grab hold of that ball of energy and to start gently pulling it down to the centre of the earth. As that happens a tube is formed, called your grounding cord, which goes from the base of your spine all the way down to the centre of the earth. Let it be good and wide, wide enough for say a football or a basketball, and let the end of it be firmly anchored into the centre of the earth, anchoring and firmly grounding you to the earth.

You should now have a flow of energy that comes from the centre of the earth, up through your feet, up your legs, into your pelvis and solar plexus (diaphragm area), then flows back down your back and into the earth through your grounding cord."

Suddenly a large tube (about 3 feet wide) connected into the base of my spine in the picture. I had a moment of panic. I had always been told to conserve my energy and now I was expected to let it go. I heard Edward's voice saying "Think of a river and remove the blocks. If the outflow is blocked the inflow will stop." With that thought the block went and all of the excess energy started pouring down my grounding chord. I could see all sorts of stuff being cleared out, I could feel in my body some of my aches and pains running along and jumping into the large tube.

"You are now connected to the earth's energy and you have done this really well and quickly, you are further developing your skill to ground and be present – not living in past events or future events, just enjoying being present. Most people have to stop and clear emotions on the way to get the flow going better.

Now I want you to notice something. Just cross your legs, please?"

As I did this the image of me on the wall crossed her legs too and the energy flow stopped almost immediately.

"Hey, what's happened?"

"Just uncross your legs and watch the energy flow restart."

"Cool."

"It may be cool, but just think what's happening to your energy every time you cross your legs and you're not grounded."

"I must miss a lot of energy!"

"Almost everyone who has dramatic energy drops for no reason is missing out on the earth's energy.

I suggest you sit there watching the picture on the wall for perhaps 5 to 10 minutes until you're quite confident you can do this yourself."

..."Great! Yes, I'm quite happy!"

"Now destroy that grounding cord and ask for another one in present time."

Now it's time for Universal Energy.[8] *Imagine way out in space there is some energy that we'll call universal energy, which is really supportive of you right now. Let it beam down towards the top of your head. As it approaches your head, it starts clearing your outer energy system, which some people call your aura; let it clean and clear your energy system until it shines on the top of your head.*

Then it starts cleaning and clearing the energy centres that are in your head. It starts travelling down the back of your neck, down your back all the way down to your pelvis. As it moves through your back it is cleaning and clearing the energy systems in all the areas of your body associated with your back.

As this energy goes into the pelvic area, it picks up some of the earth energy; you can play with the exact mixture, or let your unconscious wisdom control that.

So the universal energy from above shines on the top of your head and goes down your neck, where some of it breaks off at the level of your throat and travels through your shoulders, clearing and cleaning the energy in your shoulders, your arms, your palms and finally, let that energy shoot out of the tips of your fingers and drop down to the earth.

---

[8] Reprint from *You too can 'do' health!* page 241

All this time the rest of the universal energy continues travelling down your back to your pelvic area, picks up some earth energy and then moves up the front of your body.

As it moves up the front of your body, it cleans and clears the energy centres in the front of your body; through your abdominal cavity, chest, throat, shoulders and back up to your neck and head. It's cleaning and clearing as it moves upwards, and eventually you let it fountain back out above your head, raining down again to clean and clear your aura.

Any excess energy and cleaned out energy goes down your grounding cord and into the centre of the earth.

As these flows are working together, cleaning and clearing, imagine that your grounding cord has this wonderful ability to release anything that you are willing to let go of. Any old emotional patterns, old limiting beliefs, old mental patterns, old programming, other people's energies can just flow down through you and down your grounding cord into the centre of the earth where it gets reprocessed by the centre of the earth into positive energy.

Imagine or pretend that all three energy flows are happening very naturally, at the same time.

Take whatever time is appropriate for you to run this cleaning and clearing process. You may take 5, 10, or 15 minutes. If you only take 5 minutes a day it will change your life for the better. If you can afford to take 10 or 15 minutes, that will give you more benefit. The important thing is to give this process time on a daily basis to give you the most benefit.

And lastly, enjoy doing this energy exercise with the understanding that however long you do it for, at the end of it you will be refreshed, renewed and ready to interact with the world."

"How are you feeling?"

"Pretty amazing."

"In that case I suggest you put your hands to the floor to release any excess energy and then get up and move around, possibly have a stretch and a drink of water. And then I think that's enough for today. I'd like you to run your energy, just like this at least twice a day. Now, take a look at your energy meter again."

"It's up to 45%, and I feel a lot better. Have you got anything else to teach me?"

"Yes, but that can wait for another day."

And with that, Edward and the tree evaporated just as quickly as they had arrived.

After a few moments I got up and pottered around the house with some enjoyment, clearing up things and without feeling excessively tired.

This was great, but I wondered what the future would hold. What would I do if I got better? I would have to work. I realised I'd become so used to being ill I might not actually know how to be well.

Chapter 7: What will the future hold?

I awoke with a ping. That was the best night's sleep I had had for years. The clock said 10am and I felt really bright and alive – what day was it and what had happened? Getting out of bed I put my feet on the floor with trepidation, waiting for the normal pains to arrive. I could hear a dog barking next door and out of the window the milk cart was just clinking its way down the road.

I sat there trying to ground myself, which suddenly seemed a quite natural thing to do. My feet caught my attention, I wasn't sure why. They looked and felt different. As I gently lowered my weight onto them there wasn't any pain! Normally I would have shooting pains up my calves on the way to the bathroom. I walked a couple of steps, trying desperately to suppress my excitement in case it resulted in disappointment. Was I dreaming?

As I walked into the kitchen there was a silver fairy sitting at the kitchen table apparently having breakfast. Now I knew I must be dreaming. I walked in, put on the kettle and cleared my throat.

"Oh sorry, I've been flying all night and as you were asleep, I was sure you wouldn't mind if I helped myself to a teeny bit of toast and jam. My name is Gwendolyn by the way."

"Am I awake? Can I really be having a conversation with a fairy over the breakfast table?"

"Oh yes! You are awake, and today's a big day, this is the day you decide what your future will hold. You decide what you want."

I could feel every bone and muscle in my body recoiling at the very thought of a future. I had no idea what I wanted for my future but I was an expert on what I didn't want.

"Well," I started, "I know I don't want to be ill! I'm fed up with the way I am. I've got no friends, they drifted away years ago, I've no qualifications to do anything and I wouldn't be well enough to do any training. Is that the sort of thing you mean? It's making me feel really sad just talking about it."

"Well" said Gwendolyn, dabbing a jam spot from her chin, "You're clearly an expert on what you *don't* want. If you concentrate on what you don't want you're likely to attract even more of it. That's the Law of Attraction – we attract what we focus on, good or bad!"

"So what should I be doing?"

"Think about what you do want and how you're going to achieve it."

"But mum always says *those who want, don't get.*"

"If *you're* not focused on what you want, who else is going to be?"

"Well I don't know what I want! I've been ill so long I'm frightened of thinking about anything I want, it probably won't happen anyway and yes I know, that's another limiting belief."

"OK, OK, keep cool, just take my magic wand, and give yourself a wish. If you could be or do anything you wanted what would that be?"

"A vet. When I was little I always wanted to work with animals. But I can't possibly do that. I've no qualifications."

Gwendoline, folded her tiny silver wings with a decisive snap,

"Stay focused and dismiss all thoughts of impossibilities. What could you manage to do that would move you towards that goal?"

"Well, there's a dog down the road, I suppose I could offer to take him out for a walk to stop him barking. Oh no I couldn't! What am I thinking of? I haven't got enough energy, I'd collapse in the park."

"There you go again, an expert in what you don't want."

"I suppose I could try a shorter walk first, just around the block, and then pace myself into doing more."

"OK, Let's try 2 years from now. What would you really, really like to be doing? What would you look like, sound like and most importantly feel like?"

"Healthy...energetic...happy - have friends again."

"Great! And would you need to have a job?"

"I'd like to be training to do something, or perhaps have a part-time job."

"And what might that be?"

"Don't know, I really don't know what I can do. I've been ill since I was 14."

"There you go again, thinking about the things you can't do. Here, use my wand again and see what pictures you get this time."

Thinking this was downright crazy I took the wand again. There I was sitting in one of those metal cages that people use for dogs. A golden retriever was asleep with his head in my lap. I was stroking him. He was breathing heavily and from time to time whimpered softly. It was a huge cage and there were several others in the room, all with animals in them. It must be a vet's office. And I was wearing a green uniform.

"Hey I'm a veterinary assistant... no that can't be me, but it is! Could I really do that?"

"What do you think?"

"I don't know what qualifications you need, but I could find out."

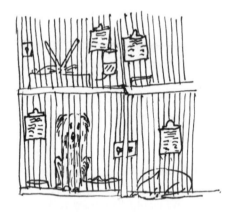

I suddenly felt energised and started off to search the internet for more information.

I turned round to thank Gwendolyn, but she was gone. All that remained was a circle of silver dust around her plate, which was spotlessly clean with a white feather on the side of it.

Sitting down in the evening, I reflected on what an interesting day it had been. I could feel myself starting to move forwards. I really liked the idea of getting out of the house and doing some kind of training even though it frightened me.

I started thinking how everything would change if I were well. There were so many unknowns that I started to panic a bit. How would I know I could do it? What would happen if I needed a rest when I was out of the house and couldn't get home again? Would anyone help me? What would the doctor say? What would my parents say? I might fail... oh this was all too overwhelming!

Chapter 8: What's been holding me stuck?

There seems to be glue all over the floor. As I walk, my whole body feels wonky, not straight, almost as if I'm drunk, with my feet dragging along the floor. I want to run but my feet won't respond. I can't see any way out, there are large boulders in the way, everywhere. I'm leaning up against a door. If this moves I'll just fall over, I haven't got the strength to do anything else. Perhaps I'd better just curl up in the corner here and hope no-one will notice. NO, I have to stand up whatever happens. There are soldiers marching past with a drill sergeant shouting "RIGHT, LEFT, RIGHT, LEFT ..."

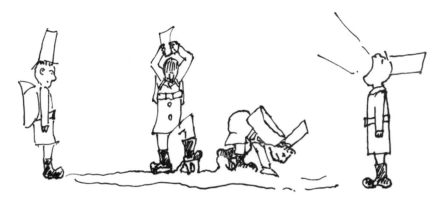

The noise is reverberating in my head whilst all this glue is holding me fast and I can't get away. There's a band coming down the street and people are dancing happily, but I can't join in. I'm still stuck and there are pools of my energy on the floor, seeping away from me in thick blue rivers. My energy is even clogging up some of the soldiers.

"Come back, come back …" but the more I shout the more tired I am and the rivers flow faster away from me … until I finally drop to the floor.

I woke up in tears. What was all that about? Another ghastly dream. Could I really move on? And the pains were back. This time my muscles seemed permanently in spasm – I could hardly move – I dragged myself to a sitting position. What was I going to do with this crippling stiffness? It was a bit like the pain I used to get at school after sports, but this was throughout my whole body as if muscles and tendons were stuck and screaming. I needed Edward; I seemed to have gone backwards.

At that moment a golden wind wafted through the window, and a sign popped up with a big question mark reminding me to ask myself how much of the energy was running my body was mine. A miserable 5% figure appeared. Now I definitely knew I was going backwards.

"Now, now, not necessarily" I heard Edward's now familiar voice with relief.

"Well how do you account for this? "

"I know you're disappointed but actually you're doing really well. Your energy didn't go down, you're simply learning what energy belongs to you, what doesn't and what was yours but is now out of date. Your meter is actually now recording closer to your energy in present time, which is the best energy for you. I just want to take you back. All those negative thoughts you generated last night plus the dreams about not being good enough and being stuck have generated more negativity, so you've blown your own fuses again."

"But," I protested, "I was so happy yesterday after talking with Gwendolyn."

"And just recall how energised that made you feel. The path to wellness has its peaks and valleys, it's not a straight line. It's all part of the process of moving forward. "

"Doesn't feel like I'm moving anywhere!" I said a bit sulkily.

"Well I'm going to teach you another technique just for fun, and this one may even make you laugh. Amusement about seeing and moving energy is always a good idea and the more fun you have the easier it will be.

But first I want to explain that being triggered like this is a great opportunity to release things you've been holding onto for some time, the events of yesterday just caused a lot of your negative stuff to bubble to the surface. Try to think of this as a present, a great opportunity to let go."

I didn't say anything but it crossed my mind that I could think of better presents. Edward though was well into his stride:

"In your dream did you recognise what the glue was about?"

"Well sometimes I feel too frightened to get well because it's a step into the unknown but at the same time most of me is desperate to get to normal!"

"That's all quite natural. It's just one of the internal conflicts you have – you surfaced a few last night when you were panicking about moving forward. When part of you wants to do one thing and part of you wants to do another or part of you gets angry and part of you hates being angry, you can manifest this internal conflict as severe pain. Why not try asking yourself how much good health you're allowed to have?"

"Really? Surely that's 100%? Never mind, I'll give it a try....Goodness, only 30%"

"This isn't surprising. We'll see how you are once you've tried this new clearing. I'm sure it will change.

You've told me several times you wish you could wash all the fuzz out of your head, well, time to give it a try and see if we can wash away some of that conflict too. I'm sure as a child you've played with those little toy people who can be taken to pieces. Head, legs, arms etc all pop off and pop on again. We're going to do the same with you. Do a scan of your body and notice how you feel now.

Just sit back and relax, put your feet on the ground and uncross your legs and arms...

This time just imagine you're taking a trip down to the edge of the lake 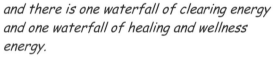 *and there is one waterfall of clearing energy and one waterfall of healing and wellness energy.*

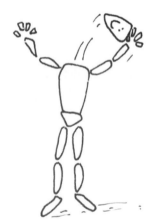

*Imagine taking your **head** off and giving it a good wash in the clearing energy, washing out any energy that isn't yours, old beliefs that limit you, old programming from other people, and old stuck emotions, Make sure it washes out all your energy channels in your head, on top of your head, in the gap between your eyebrows, where your 3rd eye*

is, all around your eyes where your sinuses run, your nose, your mouth and your teeth. Your mouth needs to be clear to take in nourishment and to communicate clearly. Be playful and don't force anything, you don't need to clear everything now. After all, you will be visiting the waterfalls often. When you have washed out everything that easily washes off (for now) transfer your head to the other waterfall, the healing and wellness energy, and let your head be energized, healed, and set at wellness and vitality. Finally reconnect it back onto your neck.

Going back to the clearing waterfall, take off your **neck**, give it a good wash in the clearing energy, letting the waterfall wash out blocks that stop you saying what you need to say. Be gentle, playful, and let the waterfall do the work.. Then transfer your neck to the healing energy waterfall and set it to wellness and vitality before putting it back in your body.

Next, take off your **arms** and repeat the process. Then take off your **legs**, your legs need to support you, in being flexible and help you to move forward. Repeat the process remembering to give them a good clean, healing and set them to wellness.

Now take out your **heart** the source of all the love you give to yourself and others. Treating it with great care and respect wash it out thoroughly in the clearing energy to let go of any negative feelings. Transfer it to the healing energy and set it to wellness, and to receiving and giving love, before returning it to your body.

Now take out your **3rd Chakra** (just below your sternum) the major source of energy in your body, imagine it opening and releasing blocks. Transfer it to the healing energy, set it to wellness and openness to your personal power and then return it to you body.

Now take out your **2nd chakra** which is a little bit below your navel, and wash out old emotions and blocks to creativity and sensuality, Take it to the healing waterfall and have it set at comfort with your emotions and creativity and return it to your body.

Now take out your **1st chakra** at the base of your spine (it has to do with your relationship to the outside, physical world) and let it be cleared of fears, limitations and anything that interferes with your relationship to the physical world. Transfer it to the healing waterfall and let it be set at a wonderful relationship with the world and return it to your body.

For wellness and vitality, you want your **internal organs** functioning well, so please take out each one of your major internal organs, one at a time, your liver, your lungs, your spleen, your thyroid, your kidneys and the adrenal glands that sit on top of them, your stomach, your bowels, your reproductive organs. Pay attention to any that you have special concerns about. You don't have to know what your internal organs look like, just be playful.. As always, transfer your internal organs to the healing waterfall where you simply set them to wellness and vitality. As you return your reproductive organs to your body attach them, with little strings, into your grounding cord – this will minimise excessive feelings of responsibility.

Now take out your immune system. It's easier to do this one as a symbol (like someone or something that protects you) or as the words **immune system** in toy blocks. Wash out the symbol or words in the clearing waterfall (including washing out allergy and food intolerance energy), and then transfer them to the healing waterfall where the immune system is set at health and wellness.

Now take out your lymph system, this is responsible for taking away all the debris from your cells. It can get overloaded from time to time, especially if you have been inactive, and it has a very subtle movement throughout your body just under the skin. It's easier to do this one as a symbol or as the words **lymph system** in toy blocks. Wash out the symbol or words in the clearing and then transfer them to the healing waterfall and set it to wellness.

Now take out all your muscles and tendons, that are responsible for keeping you mobile and flexible. It's easier to do this one as a symbol or as the words **muscles and tendons** in toy blocks. Wash out the symbol or words in the clearing and then transfer them to the healing waterfall and set it to wellness.

Now take out all the **energy channels** that route your personal energy throughout your body especially the one that you may be aware of running the entire length of your spine on the inside. Clean out your entire energy system and transfer it to healing energy and set it to wellness.

Take off your **skin**, the largest organ in your body and your boundary to the outside world, give this a good wash out, then let the healing energy run throughout it on the inside then the outside and set it to wellness, with appropriate boundaries. Then replace your skin.

Now take off your entire aura, clean it and set it to wellness and vitality.

Now recover any energy you have scattered around the world like I showed you before, clean it up and let your energy and your own essence beam down into the crown of your head.

"Notice how you feel now."

"That feels a lot better! I just want to stay here and soak this up all day."

"Take as long as you like"...

Most of my stressed muscles seemed to have relaxed which was a great relief. I thought of a few more bits to wash out as my mind drifted happily. I jumped out of that lovely state when one of those other pains shot up from my foot into my knee.

"Ow! That hurt, that's the sort of pain I get first thing in the morning."

"I have a great process specifically for shooting aches and pains. It's so simple you'll hardly believe it. But first, as soon as you put your feet on the floor in the morning, think about grounding yourself. That will be a great start. When you are asleep, people are often very ungrounded, so a few seconds of grounding is always useful in the morning.

Pain is always a message from your subconscious to tell you something isn't right. When you get these shooting pains what does it remind you of?"

"Well, they're hardly ever in the same place, so I can't tell the doctor where the problem is. It will be somewhere else in the next 10 minutes. It's as if they're sparks – a bit like a fuse box that's sparking because it has a loose connection. Powerful one minute, non-existent the next.

I watched a film recently of a major disaster where the lights and power in a building kept sparking until bits blew up and the whole thing plunged into darkness. Well, I haven't blown up yet, but I did think this reminded me of how my aches and pains rush around my body just like sparks, never in the same place."

"That's a great description. Many people suffer from this alongside fatigue. You're quite right - this is effectively a sparking in your energy system; trying to make connections and failing. Just ask yourself to make an image of whichever part of you is sparking, perhaps it's in resistance or just trying to attract your attention."

"It certainly does that!"

"Have you got an image for the part sparking? You can have any image you like. Many people would use a rose."

"I've got a dried out sink! Is that OK?"

"Excellent and quite original. Now ask your dried out sink to look down at the ground, accept and enjoy the earth's energy, then look up and accept and enjoy Universal energy."

"Hey, this is excellent! It loves all this energy and is really clean, happy and glowing now. Not sure how I know a sink is happy, but still..."

"Now ask to take any learning from this situation that you need. Even if you're not conscious of what this is, just asking the question will be enough. Then ground the sink right down into the centre of the earth and watch it disappear."

"That was fantastic! The pain just disappeared too!"

"You see, this was a part of you that didn't have enough energy, hence the sparking. You simply acknowledged it, energised it, took any learning you needed and let it go. It is also a good idea to fill up with golden energy as usual after that."

"I'll try it on a few more and see what happens..."

Each time the pain just vanished, as if by magic.

"How does your energy feel now?"

"Much better. About 30%. But how often do I need to keep doing this sort of stuff?"

"It may feel like a full time job at the moment. That's just to get you more conscious of what's happening and clear out the backlog of energy that's been blocking your body for years. I would recommend you spend 15 minutes morning and evening clearing your energy. You'll soon find out what is the right time for you and that may be different from day to day.

Just like washing, sometimes you need a bath, other days just a quick shower may be enough, only you will know how much time you need to spend, and even 5 minutes a day would make a positive difference. You can use any of the skills I've taught you and change the metaphors to suit yourself. Clearing other energies will give you more of your own energy to return to wellness. And how much health are you allowed to have now?"

"A full 80%! How did that happen?"

"More than likely you've just released some of those limiting beliefs, metaphors etc that you've been associating with illness. They'll have been stored in the cells of your body. Now they've gone, gone for good and you've been resetting your body to wellness. Now you'll find it a lot easier to regain your health."

"I really have lost the deep feeling that I need to be unwell. I can't get it back however hard I try."

"It's great to know it's gone and you don't have to try any more to have the feeling. It has left you.

It's time for you to have fun. Life is supposed to be fun!"

With that Edward took himself off disappeared in a golden puff of smoke.

Chapter 9: Maisey has an idea

I was just going to make myself some lunch when I noticed Maisey was sitting at the table too. I must have looked startled, because there spread out in front of her on the table was a really healthy looking lunch, seemingly arrived from no-where.

"Don't mind me my dear," she said, filling her plate with some interesting choices. "I just dropped in to help you with what you said about putting on too much weight. Can you elaborate?"

"Sometimes I eat and eat and still want more. I never feel full or satisfied. It's often when I've had a bit of an upset or after a difficult phone call. Often late in the day too. I know I shouldn't do it but I just can't seem to stop it. No self control and if I start eating chocolate, I have to finish the whole bar."

"And you'd like all this to change?"

"Absolutely, but I've been doing it for such a long time. Can I really get unstuck from this one too? Actually I normally eat quit well, and when I have these eating binges it's like it's not really me in control."

"Probably isn't." Said Maisey, daintily wielding her own knife and fork and speaking politely between mouthfuls.

"The energy for overeating can be attached to emotions, so if you feel frustrated, it may well go back to a time when you *were* frustrated and to what you were told about food when you were very little."

"Into my head pops a familiar phrase, *Eat up now, we can't afford to waste food, other people in the world are starving.*"

Maisey nodded,

"That's exactly what I mean. But carrying those beliefs around with you now is only going to make you overeat when a similar emotion is triggered."

"And what about *if you don't finish your food you won't have any energy.* That one's still being used - telling me to eat more to get more energy."

"And how's it working?"

"Dreadfully – the more food I eat, the more weight I put on and the more tired I get."

"So let's try something. Can you try blowing up those beliefs one at a time? They may have been useful some time ago but they're not serving you well today".

"You're right, they're well past their sell by date and I'm only too happy to get rid of them. There they go, one at a time exploded!"

"Now I'd like you to drink some water, clear your energy for just 5 minutes then get in touch with how hungry you really are."

As I cleared my energy I saw all sorts of stuff heading off to the lake. Maisey was smiling in approval,

"Excellent, now just fill up with gold energy again, gold energy will help you feel more like you and it's food for your energy system. It doesn't need you to fill up with physical food too."

Feeling lighter already, I looked at the delicious spread on the table.

"Just concentrate on how hungry you are and if you're thirsty take a drink first, sometimes people get hunger and thirst confused. Select what you'd like and put it on that lovely clean plate. It really is important you're free to choose what you'd like to eat. Nobody makes progress eating what they don't like. And I want you to make it look attractive on that plate, don't just throw it on like a snack out of the fridge."

I made myself up a lovely plate of salad, hummus, fresh, still-warm French bread, soup and some yoghurt. It looked and smelt great. As I started to eat Maisey admonished,

"Slowly, eat consciously, savour every mouthful and chew it well. Don't forget you can leave some if you've taken too much. Enjoy your lunch," and she popped one last radish from her plate into her mouth, picked up her bag and disappeared.

I was about half way through lunch when I noticed I was feeling full. That was something I hadn't noticed till too late for years, by which time I usually felt bloated. I put down my cutlery and looked at what was left on the plate. I no longer felt I had to finish, so I cleared away and congratulated myself on accepting some really good ideas to start me on a healthier lifestyle. Maisey really is a great detective, I thought.

That afternoon I felt really strong. I left the house and walked to the park without a second thought.

Chapter 10: Clowning around

It was Sunday afternoon, kids were playing, dogs were running around and on the lake were ducks and swans. The spring sun was warm on the top of my head and as I walked I could feel it entering my body, and energy running through my veins. I couldn't remember when I'd last felt like this.

In the distance I could see a clown entertaining a group of children seated around him on the grass. Well, the kids were actually falling around laughing. When was the last time I laughed? I couldn't remember.

My legs started taking me in the direction of the clown, I didn't seem to be quite in control of my direction any more.

The clown beckoned to me to sit down with the children. Their laughter was infectious. They were giggling at the clown, with the helpless laughter that grabs us when we're small. I could feel a giggle bubbling up in me too. I didn't know what I was laughing at, maybe it was just infectious.

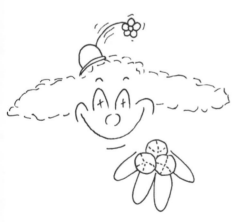

When I looked up at the clown he was pulling silly faces. He didn't care how stupid he looked. He was trying to juggle and everything went wrong. He and the audience were having a ball.

I suddenly realised it was OK to make mistakes and a great skill to be able to laugh at yourself. At that moment the clown ran over, gave me a set of juggling balls and got me to join in.

I had never juggled and couldn't get the hang of it. The more mistakes I made, the more I laughed and the more the children laughed. For the first time in my life mistakes didn't matter. And then a really strange thing happened. Between tears of laughter, I suddenly started juggling and over the next 10 minutes I got better and better and the children cheered me on. Not only was I a success but I was having fun.

The kids were shouting:

"Good one!"

"You're the best!"

"What a star!"

I must have been there for 30 minutes until the end of the show; in fact I was part of the show. I'd laughed so much my belly ached and I was so happy that walking back home later I felt as if I was walking on air. I was tired, but this was a different sort of tiredness, this was good tiredness.

After dinner, I ran my energy just like Edward had showed me. It seemed to come up from the earth much more easily; I could feel it tingling through my body and happily running down my grounding cord. I was relaxed and enjoyed the feeling. I was still smiling about the children and the clown in the park when I went to bed.

Curling up in my bed, I found my arms wrapped around my teddy bear, Bongo. He had a really kind face. He'd been with me through thick and thin since I was just 6 months old. As I looked into his face, he said,

"Excuse me, I have been meaning to have a word."

"About?" I replied as if conversation with a bear was quite normal.

"About you protecting yourself."

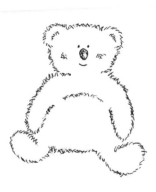

"From what?"

"All that negative energy you're sensitive to. You have been picking it up all your life and it exhausts you."

"How do you know that?"

"We bears are pretty sharp you know. And I have been around a long time. When you were very little you used to hug me lots and I often helped protect you, but once you got older I didn't get so many hugs and you didn't get so much protection.

You know Edward was telling you all that stuff about meridians and chakras; well your chakras have always been open, so I think it's time I taught you about how to protect yourself. You can't carry me or a cushion around with you all day, now you're an adult."

"I'm not sure I understand?"

"It's easy! Just imagine when you're talking to someone, there's a small teddy bear grounded into the earth between you and the other person. Imagine talking to the bear, rather than the other person directly.

You don't want to put your energy into their space, nor accept their energy into yours.

The teddy bear keeps your energies separate so you won't be so affected. If you didn't want to go with a teddy, you can do the same thing with a rose, or any other object. Just remember, make sure it's fully grounded, so the energy slips back into the earth.

Now you're more aware of energies you'll probably notice any negativity you want to avoid. You can always choose to imagine it bouncing off the outside of your aura and you can visualise your chakras closing (like a camera lens) to avoid energies you don't want. That's great! I can see you're getting the idea already. Some people really drain your energy, like the woman next door."

"Goodness me, what makes you say that?"

"Oh, I've heard her telling you how dreadful things are. I know you like company, but she makes you even more tired. Although you could also try imagining you're surrounded by a shell of invisible but semi-permeable golden light, like wrapping yourself in a giant egg. I used to do that when you and your brother used to throw me around. I never got hurt in my egg. You can adjust your level of protection depending on the circumstances. If you know you're going to be in a difficult situation just increase your level of protection."

"Thanks. That's really helpful, and I feel so guilty because I can really remember you being thrown across the room by Tom and me."

"Just one more thing. Don't watch any negative films until you're really good at protection. I can feel negativity coming from the TV and from you when you hug me and it really jangles me, let alone the effect it has on you."

"I always knew you were a fabulous bear who'd take care of me."

At that moment I saw a handful of beautifully coloured balloons appearing. Some had words written on them like "fun", "love", "gratitude", "joy", "appreciation", "forgiveness", "care", "judgement free".

"Pick whichever ones you like as a present to nourish your heart and wellbeing"

As I selected the lovely pink, yellow and orange ones I could feel a glow in my heart that radiated throughout my body.

"This is wonderful, thank you so much. Sleep tight Bongo."

Chapter 11: Releasing unwanted memories

That dog down the road woke me up again. Why don't they take him out for a walk and why does he keep waking me? It seems to be happening every day.

Wait a moment; I saw a article yesterday, *Everything Happens For A Reason* so "WHY IS THAT DOG BARKING? AND AM I MAKING THIS HAPPEN?"

I didn't think that was the case, but the article was pretty categoric. It pointed out if you don't take notice and resolve the situation, the same thing or similar will keep happening.

Am I meant to offer to... surely not, you can't just pitch up at someone's front door and offer to walk their dog, can you? On the other hand - nothing ventured, nothing gained.

But what if it was a horrible aggressive dog and the owner might be pretty aggressive too. An image of Gwendolyn suddenly popped into my head. "Nothing," she pointed out sharply, "Ventured, nothing gained!"

And so I found myself knocking on the door of a complete stranger. A little old lady answered looking apprehensive. I introduced myself, said I was going down to the park, would she like me to take her dog for a walk.

I could hear my internal voice murmuring, "Are you nuts?" but I ignored it. The lady was thrilled, told me she was unable to take Bonnie out herself and had had no-one to help since her husband died a few months ago.

Bonnie was cute. She came and sniffed all around me, as if doing an inspection. I was certainly being interviewed. She finally wagged her tail and the deal was done. She swaggered down the road, waited at the crossroad and seemed really happy to meet other dogs. I sat down on a bench and she sat down next to me, like a sentry on guard. I heard "Open your chakras and enjoy the sunshine."

I glanced at Bonnie, she winked! "I mean it, open your chakras and we can enjoy the sunshine together. What a lovely day you've picked. I'm terribly appreciative of you taking me out."

So I sat there enjoying the sunshine with what seemed to be my own, newly acquired but extremely polite personal body guard. I found I could open my chakras, receive more energy and close them again, just by thinking about it. And the more I appreciated what I'd achieved in the last few days the better and calmer I felt.

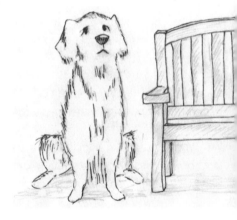

Bonnie started telling me her story of how upset she had been when her master died. She had been with him when he collapsed. When the ambulance came, they didn't know where to take her so she'd ended up at the police station. She dreams about it most nights so in the morning, she just wants to go out for a walk and forget it, that's why she barks.

As I listened to her story I recalled also getting lost – as a youngster. I strayed from my mother in a shopping mall and was taken to the office so they could make a lost child announcement. I could still vividly remember it and like Bonnie, my story didn't seem to have an end; my memory just stopped when I was lost, giving me the feeling that nobody cared about me either. Somehow I just didn't deserve to be here. Maybe that is where some of my negative beliefs have come from

Sitting down on the grass, I helped Bonnie change her story round and realise she had eventually got home safely. I reminded her how much her Mum loved her but was too old now to take her for walks and I asked her to imagine her master was now in heaven and having a fun time. I offered to come around as often as I could and we'd take lovely walks together. Bonnie leant over and licked my hand. "Thank you so much," she said. "That would be just delightful." [9]

And while helping Bonnie, I changed my story too. Because I could clearly see my Mum come up to me and give me the world's biggest hug. So I didn't need to feel lonely any more. And as I said that to Bonnie I saw loads of old memories disappearing to the magnet in the lake; I must have released some really good stuff this time.

At that moment an Irish Setter called Magnum came bounding over to Bonnie and they started leaping about happily on the grass. I looked up and saw Magnum's owner smiling at me – neither of us needed to be lonely any more.

Walking back home, several things had changed within me and I knew things were *looking up.* I had had a great chat with Magnum's owner. He knew Bonnie and was delighted to see her out and about again. He'd wondered what had happened to her, but didn't know where she lived so hadn't been able to find out any more about her. Magnum and Bonnie had been old friends. They were delighted to meet again.

---

[9] If you have traumatic memories to release, an NLP practitioner can help you very quickly, which will make releasing negative energy much more effective. Please contact the author for any further assistance.

Chapter 12: A compelling future

As I was walking back up the front garden again, everything seemed different. Things were certainly **looking up**. It was a glorious spring day, the sun was shining and I could feel it boosting my energy system.

Just a minute! There was Gwendolyn curled up in a corner of the settee, looking as if she'd been having a nap.

"I see you've had a great day."

"Certainly have and I'm feeling much more positive about looking at the future. What a coincidence you're here now!"

"Um, synchronicity is much more than just a coincidence. We just attract things and people into our lives when we most need them, to either learn from or to help us take the next step forward. The more we notice synchronicities, the more they happen."[10]

"I've been moving forward all day."

"Now it's time to really focus on what you want and how you're going to achieve it."

"Taking Bonnie out for a walk seemed a huge step, but it was actually so easy and Mrs Potts was thrilled I'd offered."

"So what's the next step?"

---

[10] Deepak Chopra, Synchrodestiny

"That mind's eye picture of sitting in the dog's cage with a Golden Retriever. It gives me a real buzz and a glow in my heart. Do you think I can do it?"

"Well you won't know until you have a go. Why don't you see what it would be like. Take my wand and magic up another you about 3 feet away. Take a good look at that woman, she's about 3 years older than you are now. What does she look like? What's she wearing? What's her hair like? The expression on her face? What's she saying, feeling, thinking? What might other people be saying about her? Just try walking forward into that space and see what it feels, looks and sounds like. You can always step out of it if you don't like it and change the image."

As I walked forward, all the colours became brighter and I felt more and more excited. This was all feeling really possible for the first time in my life, nothing was holding me back any more. All I needed to do was take more steps along the journey. I could see a staircase and me smiling with every new step I climbed.

"I can do this and I do have a future. Keeping this image in mind is going to pull me towards it. I have this warm glow throughout my body. I feel this is so right and I have a plan."

"Clasp your hands together and connect to that feeling. That's great! You now have an anchor to that feeling, so whenever you clasp your hands together you can get it back again."

This was really exciting. When I thought of the pile of washing up in the kitchen the feeling went, so I just clasped my hands together and whoosh! The feeling of having a great future was back with me.

Chapter 13: Reviewing my journey

"Now go backwards and just consider what was keeping you stuck and sick when you first met the green goblin."

"I can see a pattern emerging. When it all started, I was very busy, extremely stressed – a new school, a couple of really negative friends and I caught a virus from which my energy system didn't recover.

Once I became so used to being ill it was scary to consider what it would be like to be well. Through my illness I'd really missed out on being a teenager and didn't think I knew how to be an adult. Every time I tried to move forward I picked up more negative energy and that knocked me back again.

I have so many thoughts flying around in my head when you ask that question, that first of all I will focus on being grounded, put them into groups and try to assemble a coherent answer.

I needed to clear up some things from the past, and this journey has taught me:

√   To release energetic blocks

√   Let go of stuff I no longer need, including traumatic events.

√   Inspect and change beliefs that were inappropriate and probably out of date.

√   Clear my energy.

√   Recover my energy from wherever I've scattered it - this made me instantly feel a lot stronger and complete.

√ Ground myself so I can access the earth's energy and release those emotions that had stopped me grounding. Also to ground some of those overwhelming responsibilities.

√ Listen to my own internal dialogue and ensure the metaphors I use are positive.

√ Take notice of that holiday experience, remember the time I recovered all my energy on holiday and lost it again when I came home; that was trying to tell me something and I lost the opportunity by ignoring it."

"Excellent! " Gwendoline clapped her hands with delight.

"You've cleared a lot but you mustn't forget your regular daily routine. Also remember when something or someone **presses your buttons** it's not their fault, but it's your opportunity to do more clearing.

In my mind I could see Maisey's face grinning from ear to ear.

"Now you understand what happened you can be in control again."

"I needed to understand more to help me:

√ Become aware of my energy system, how to look after it and exclude the energy of others. Within my aura my own energy is senior to other peoples'.

√ Reduce my emotional response and thus reduce stress, so my fuses don't blow.

√ See that although I thought I was committed to getting well, there were parts of me seeing myself as a sick person. The guided imagery helped me clear those beliefs.

√ Start a step by step programme of moving forward with a little exercise and a good diet.

√ Give and receive love and companionship, even from unlikely sources.

√ Reading *You too can 'do' health!* filled in many areas of knowledge for me.

√ Have more fun and laughter – laughing broke up my miserable feelings, giving me positive energy.

√ Appreciate myself and what I'm achieving."

"Great! This is all about becoming more self aware and committed to what you want rather than what you don't want."

"And to move into the future, probably the most important factors for me were:

√ Finding a compelling future – an essential part of healing although it had always been the last thing on my mind.

√ Being more connected with my body. Acknowledging rather than ignoring my own wisdom.

√ Curiosity – being curious about daily events and seizing opportunity.

√ Seeing that staircase I knew I could climb albeit slowly. I learnt the doctor's message all those years ago was probably right even though poorly delivered.

√ Feeling my immune system change and focus. I'm now confident the food intolerances will diminish.

√   A strategy for the future – I have the tools so if I have a dip of energy again, I know exactly what to do about it.

√   Knowing the more I love Bonnie, the more I love myself. I'm ready to bring people to love back into my life."

"This is an excellent resume and although everyone experiences different sets of symptoms, underlying causes are the same, UNDERSTANDING YOUR ENERGY SYSTEM AND LEARNING TO KEEP IT HEALTHY.

I thought about that for a moment, then nodded my head in agreement,

"Yes, it was definitely an ENERGY DISTRIBUTION ISSUE, once my energy was flowing I lost that drained feeling, all my lights came back on. The aches and pains were calls for help from different parts of me and once supplied with energy, I took the learning and the messages stopped. Also releasing anger and frustration let go all that tension and stress in my muscles."

I've also learned how open I was to negative energy. I remember my mother saying what a 'sensitive child' I was.

 I know now it's OK to have emotions but not be consumed by them and to protect myself by clearing out negative ones."

"So," said Gwendoline, "What were the secondary benefits you were getting from illness?"

"Glad you left that one till last. I guess I was getting some benefit or I wouldn't have had the problem.

Let me see. I suppose it stopped me being so busy, and I sort of enjoyed that. I'd always felt I should spend my life doing everything for everyone else but this made me focus on me. Odd isn't it that Myalgic Encephalomyelitis has the initials ME?

But now I have found my passion in life, what I really want to do, I've taken the first steps and I'm thrilled with the goal. I feel as if all the jigsaw pieces of my life are coming together at last.

I also have the guided imagery which I can utilise whenever I need.

I 'm not sure I've found all the reasons for being stuck. I think they will emerge over the next few months and years, but I'm now focused on being free to follow my passion, I have a plan, my own resources and I am smiling!"

With that Gwendolyn flew up, wrapped her wings around me for one last hug and was off, with just a trail of fairy dust.

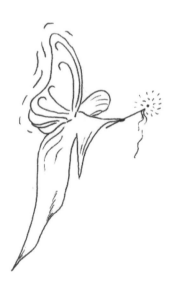

Personal stories

Helen's story

I have suffered with fatigue for twenty years and was diagnosed with ME in 1995. You were the last step in helping me to get rid of the ME/Chronic Fatigue I have been suffering from. I've been getting better slowly over the years but never seemed to be able to get over the pain I kept feeling in my legs and every time I exercised I would get ill and it would take me months to recover. I am now able to run, walk up stairs and do many things without the pain and the debilitating tiredness. You have helped me run my energy and got rid of the blockages I had in my legs, plus the grounding of my internal female organs. I would never have believed, just by doing that alone, I no longer have this constant feeling of responsibility and drain I had been feeling before. That alone made such a difference to the way I felt. Then, when I learnt to put my feet on the ground and became grounded, well I haven't looked back. I have no pain in my legs and I can't even remember what it felt like now! I can run up many, many stairs and nothing happens. I haven't been able to do that since I was in my teens. Thank you Olive for your direction and time.

Katherine's story

Thank you so much for the gift you have given me:

I have been able to fast track my recovery from ME thanks to the wonderful skills you have taught me in clearing my energy and through reading this book and reaffirming the skills you have taught me on a regular basis. I highly recommend anyone who thinks that they have

ME or chronic fatigue to enlist your services and start their journey to a full recovery. Your book is wonderful - it takes us on a journey of discovery, following the path to good health, removing stuck energy and making us aware of how powerful our subconscious mind is. Many thanks for the wonderful work you do.

Penny's story

I was diagnosed in 2003 with MS after a long period in hospital. I was given physiotherapy and occupational therapy as my support when I came out of hospital but these all focused on the illness and not the getting better. One of the focuses was on fatigue management and I wanted to work on recovering my energy not on fatigue that was holding me back. When I discovered Energetic NLP it was a lifesaver. It focuses on knowing what is your energy and how to recover it. I haven't looked back since. This book offers people with MS a really easy way to get back in control of their energy and then who knows what they might achieve. My life path completely changed when I was diagnosed with MS, as you can imagine, but now it has changed again and so much for the better. I know I've got more energy now than even before the MS. Penny, Hertfordshire

Postscript from Olive Hickmott

I am delighted you have completed the healing story part of this book and trust you found it beneficial in your journey to wellness. I will be thrilled to receive your feedback, especially if I can publish it to assist others.

For me, putting an energy perspective on top of my Neuro-linguistic Programming (NLP) training made perfect sense and filled a gap which I'd been aware existed both for my health clients and for myself. But the really great thing about EnergeticNLP is that it's so available and simple to learn, even for people who've done little or no personal development or training such as NLP.

"Energy matters" is one of those expressions I use frequently. Your personal energy matters a great deal to your health, to achieving your goals and in all other aspects of your life. It's something most of us take for granted, until we're faced with having little or no energy and may even have developed Chronic Fatigue.

Art Giser[11], developer of EnergeticNLP and my teacher, is simply a master at teaching you the simple skills you can use to manage your own energy. If you look at the complementary therapies, almost all are focused on enabling your energy to flow smoothly throughout your body, whether it is EFT, Massage, Reflexology, Qigong or a host of others. "If your energy is flowing freely you will be healthy". One of the best things about EnergeticNLP is that anyone and everyone can easily learn the skills needed. Once learnt they are skills for life, for

---

[11] Art Giser, www.energeticNLP.com

health and for enjoyment and you'll soon be able to do these processes on your own using them anytime and anywhere.

So EnergeticNLP at one level is a simple tool for anyone to gain control of energy flow through their body to achieve maximum health, wellbeing and so much more. If we'd been brought up in an Eastern culture, understanding personal energy would be commonplace. It takes just a few minutes a day to practice, soon becoming part of your daily routine. Other levels of EnergeticNLP offer other processes to release negative emotions that are not covered in this book and so much more, to develop every aspect of healing you could wish for, for yourself and your clients.

At my business, Empowering Health, lack of energy is treated very seriously, it is very real. However, with 3-4 coaching sessions in person or over the telephone, someone who is committed to succeeding can be taught the tools and processes to recover that energy and return to wellness.

This book is an essential starter in your journey and through the skills available at Empowering Health other personalised processes can be used. Training programmes are available to teach you all the skills you need:

- √ The New Perspectives technique to overcome ME, Chronic Fatigue, etc as described in this book, Recover your energy, and including any further developments post publication.
- √ EnergeticNLP: an introduction for local communities and therapist groups and the full level 1 or level 2 trainings (see www.energeticNLP.co.uk)
- √ The Empowering Health Coaching structure for great results.

For those who want to learn more about EnergeticNLP programmes, far exceeding material covered in this book, they are available in the USA, UK and several other countries. Take a look at Art Giser's web-site is www.energeticNLP.com. Empowering Health sponsors the UK programmes that can be found on www.energeticNLP.co.uk.

You will notice that in my map of the world the client has to do all the work, guided by the coach either personally or on the phone. For some people all they need for a return to wellness is this book and where possible, the accompanying CD. We teach the tools to sustain progress hence the name *Empowering Health*.

We teach clients to:
1   Understand their own personal energy system
2   Release energetic blocks that can be painful
3   Listen to their bodies, measuring energy and seeking causes for the lack of it.
4   Reduce excessive feelings of responsibility
5   Detect the difference between their energy and others.
6   Move forward to a future that draws them.

My firm belief is everyone should have access to this knowledge, and in a way everyone can understand, simply a gift that you accept, reject or modify according to your needs.

And of course, when we've been ill throughout our young lives, this causes challenges about who we will be when we recover our health.

This New Perspectives project is ongoing as new clients and feedback will always further our knowledge. As you know, I'm committed to making any new knowledge freely available and I'm looking to publish a healing story for very young children.

This book is designed to educate you on the causes of fatigue and as greater understanding is achieved, you may feel some deep emotions that trigger negative energy. If you are unable to clear these emotions seek out an NLP Practitioner or better still one of the growing group of EnergeticNLP practitioners worldwide, that I would be pleased to put you in contact with. In this way you can simply and quickly clear the emotions troubling you

This book runs in parallel with, the earlier book *You too can 'do' health!* and the *Energetic NLP in 10 minutes per day* audio CD.

You too can 'do' health! is number 2 in the New Perspectives series. Written for everyone to understand *You too can 'do' health!* tells a great story, whilst demystifying the jargon often associated with personal development. We can all positively affect our own health with a few, how to's. *You too can 'do' health!* is the story of one person's journey of self development and awareness, as an inspiration to start your own journey. Using the tools of NLP, universal energy and the secret law of attraction, achieve the health and well-being you want. We have daily testimonials about the positive effects of this book on people's health. People report how they take from it what they need at any particular time and often re-reading triggers more and new insights.

EnergeticNLP in 10 minutes per day, and audio CD, includes an introduction to EnergeticNLP and a number of guided imagery meditations.

The difference is that this book, *Recover your energy*, is totally focused on recovering your energy and wellness from fatigue, and the web-site offers a CD which is designed specifically for this book, with all the guided meditations and additional valuable information.

Postscript: Please be aware that one of the causes of fatigue can be the negativity caused by poor literacy skills. The effort people put in to trying to spell and read plus the bullying they are often subject to can be enough to generate so much negativity that it seriously affects their energy levels and causes destructive confusion in the front of the brain. My first New Perspectives book, Seeing Spells Achieving enables people to overcome this confusion. If you would like to know more about this do take a look at www.empoweringlearning.co.uk.

My Story – a different version of pain and fatigue

I had my own experience of being really tired at University – I'd gone through a high stress situation and was diagnosed as suffering from glandular fever – a convenient label as I'd never had a positive blood test. I thought I'd recovered but memories of that tiredness stayed with me. And then I developed increasingly painful shooting sensations in my legs and lower abdomen and shortly afterward suffered a ruptured appendix with a 2 week hospital stay.

By now I was fatigued and the pains were worse. My surgical wounds were slow to heal and I knew my abdominal energy was stuck and then I started blowing up electrical equipment – two printers in 24 hours, followed by my computer a few days later – I knew I was in trouble - my energy was all wrong, but I had no idea how I could change it.

So my own journey to personal energy began, but being a health and wellness coach with skills to help people with all sorts of health challenges I now appreciated there was so much more I needed to learn.

The simple techniques of EnergeticNLP and my own personal growth have enabled me to recover my personal energy, mend all the fuses and teach others to do this for themselves. I call myself a health, wellness and energy coach but actually believe I'm an educator, committed to helping others take responsibility for their own health by finding them the tools and skills they need.

I owe a huge debt of gratitude to Art Giser, who has brought together the best of NLP and the best of energetic healing systems over the last 24 years to create EnergeticNLP. He made it easy for people like me to access these tools for themselves and to assist others and coached me through the process of developing *Recover your energy*.

Further assistance for you and others

There are a number of ways that you can access further assistance.

I offer coaching and workshop services through my health practice www.empoweringhealth.co.uk where you will see further information about EnergeticNLP and the latest findings of the project. I can offer you contact details for those I have trained.

I can be contacted at olive@empoweringhealth.co.uk

www.empoweringhealth.co.uk is part of the www.thehickmottpartnership.co.uk

There is also a CD available from www.empoweringhealth.co.uk for anyone who would like to be guided through some of the material in *Recover your energy*. The contents are:

√ all the guided imagery meditations

√ individual stories

√ processes and questions for you to think about, e.g. "What would life be like if I were better?"

√ self-help queries such as How did YOU feel? What came into YOUR mind? What insights have YOU had?

√ additional bonus tracks from Art Giser

√ information about the project.

If you are interested in working to help others I run a training programme to teach Health Coaching, including the New Perspectives

Chronic Fatigue recovery process. There are more details of this on the web-site.

If you need any help to achieve what is described in this book, you are welcome to contact me for assistance. Training courses are run for those who wish to work with others. Dates are available on the web-site.

If there is anything traumatic about the way a belief was formed, you may need to deal with this in person with an NLP Practitioner. Traumas don't have to be life threatening. An NLP practitioner can help you to change this state using the NLP trauma process and then you will be able to simply release the energy from this event.

~~~

Glossary

Allergy: The physiological equivalent of a phobia, a rapid or repeated overreaction to a specific stimulus on the part of the immune system. An allergy is an inappropriate reaction to something that is not life threatening in itself.

Anchor: An anchor makes it easier for you to recall an event, a feeling, a picture, a sound or several at once. Music often gives you a great anchor for recalling past events.

Aura: The energetic field that surrounds each living thing: Often described as egg shaped and frequently said to be different colours depending on the state of health.

Beliefs: What you take as true. The generalisations one makes about ourselves, others and the universe.

Being present: Not focused on past concerns or future worries, being present with your experience in the moment.

Chakra: Major energy centres

Confusion: A state you are in when you are struggling to achieve what you want. It is a natural feeling when we learn something new.

Conscious: Anything you are currently aware of.

Energy Field: Everyone has one. The bubble of light, sound, feelings, energy that surrounds each person.

Exhaustion and Fatigue: "Fatigue is the absence of physical, intellectual, and emotional energy, and chronic fatigue is a prolonged absence of this energy."[12] Some people use the expression exhaustion. For consistency fatigue has been used throughout this book.

Framing: When you change the frame around a picture, let's say from brown to red, the picture can take on a different look or feel as other colours are highlighted. Framing is the way you label your experiences to give them meaning. Simply by changing the frame (re-framing) you can change the meaning of your experience and see things very differently.

Grounded: Feeling as if you are firmly connected to the ground, focused. Grounding balances and centres your body and allows you to feel safer, clearer and more supported. Recall seeing a gymnast land on the floor, really firmly, or when someone is doing yoga and standing on one leg.

Lighting up: A state in your energy field when you are reacting to current circumstances and emotions.

'Mind's eye': The mental picture you paint of an object or word that you can see by recalling that image from your memory.

Programming: We are all programmed by others from a very young age. Our parents programme us not to run out in the road without looking for example. However we also pick up negative programming as well.

Re-framing: Changing your way of understanding a statement or behaviour to give it another meaning; changing the frame. The ability to reframe allows you to make sense of events that have previously been

---

[12] Boundless Energy, Deepak Chopra, Perfect Health Library

difficult or impossible in ways that work for you and create desirable emotional states.

Resources: Anything you notice or need that will assist you to hold a state.

State: Simply how you are at any one time.

Strategy: The way you do something and the process you use time and again for doing it – some work well, but others do not.

Subconscious: Everything that is not in your current awareness.

Trigger: An event or circumstance that triggers an emotion.

Visualisation: The process of capturing and holding a mental image or photograph.

Bibliography and Resources

Some of these books are referred to directly in this book whilst others are interesting background reading to further your experience in a particular area of the material covered.

Childre, doc and Martin, Howard, *The Heartmath Solution*, Harper Collins, 2000

Chopra, Deepak, *Synchrodestiny: Harnessing the Infinite Power of Coincidence to Create Miracles*, Random House Group, 2003

Chopra, Deepak, *Boundless* Energy, Random House Group, 1995

Dilts, Robert. *Changing Beliefs*, Meta Publications, 1990

Dilts, Robert, Hallbom, Tim, and Smith, Suzi. *Beliefs: Pathways to Health and Well-being*, Metamorphous Press, 1990

Friedlander, John, Hemsher, Gloria, *Basic Psychic Development*, Weiser Books, 1999

Galgano, Tianna, *Decipher your dreams, decipher your life*, Dream On Creations, 2003

Griffin, Joe and Tyrrell, Ivan, *Dreaming Reality*, HG Publishing, 2004

Mckenna, Paul, *I can make you think*, Bantam Press, 2005

McTaggart, Lynn, *The Intention Experiment*, Harper Element, 2008 and *The Field*, Harper Collins, 2001

West, Thomas G., *In the Mind's Eye*, Prometheus Books, 1997

Appendix 1: What is fatigue?

This section has been prepared by my colleague Diana Kingham to provide a summary of some of the medical knowledge and existing approaches to the treatment of fatigue. This is aimed at medical and complementary practitioners, and those with fatigue who would like to know more.

What is fatigue?

All around us we see nature and our physical environment abounding with energy. Most children take their energy for granted. So why is it that fatigue (exhaustion, extreme tiredness or lack of energy) is something most of us have experienced at one time or another? Possibly up to 25% of the population experience fatigue at any one time.

Fatigue is a common health complaint and also one of the hardest to define – it is usually taken to mean feeling tired, weak, exhausted, having a lack of energy and motivation. It is a symptom (rather than a specific disease or disorder) that can result from many different medical conditions. It can be either mental or physical (or both) in origin and is often difficult to treat by conventional approaches to health.

Any type of fatigue can indicate a serious medical condition and needs prompt medical investigation. Fatigue can make it difficult for you to perform ordinary tasks. It affects everyone differently; you may feel very tired and all you want to do is sleep, it may feel like you are wading through treacle or as if your brain is packed in cotton wool soaked in anaesthetic (this is how I remember it). It may also be accompanied by pain and sometimes can make you feel that you have little control over your life. In many cases, exercise and repeated activity will build up strength and stamina and the fatigue will disappear. In other cases this is positively counterproductive.

How is fatigue diagnosed?

Typically when you have persistent fatigue, your doctor will review your symptoms and ask about your daily routine, work habits and environmental conditions. He or she will give you a physical examination and may want you to have basic blood tests to rule out diseases that may cause fatigue. If you are under a lot of emotional stress or experience recurrent anxiety or depression, your doctor may diagnose fatigue caused by psychological disturbances.

Chronic Fatigue is diagnosed normally by exclusion when the standard blood tests come back negative and other serious illnesses have been eliminated.

What causes fatigue?

Fatigue may be physical or mental in its origin and has a huge number of possible underlying causes. You may have physical fatigue as the result of a long day of hard work or a hectic schedule. In contrast, emotional fatigue maybe more striking in the morning and less draining as the day progresses. Fatigue may also apparently come from nowhere to suddenly overwhelm you.

Many medical conditions may have associated fatigue, including: MS (Multiple Sclerosis), Cancer, Anaemia, Hepatitis, Rheumatoid Arthritis, Hypothyroidism (under-active thyroid) and Glandular Fever.

Some other causes of physical fatigue include: Infections such as Influenza; lack of sleep, poor physical condition, lack of exercise, obesity or pregnancy; environmental sources, for example, exposure to chemicals, such as pesticides and formaldehyde; side effects of certain prescription and over-the-counter medications such as antihistamines and blood pressure medications; medical treatments such as surgery, chemotherapy and radiotherapy; and chronic pain.

Some causes of emotional fatigue include: depression, anxiety, overextending yourself, trying to hide your emotions from other, major life change and stress

The category that has not hitherto been identified is energetic fatigue, for example: the result of a person of being sensitive to negative emotions, taking on other people's problems or being adversely affected by bad news.

CFS/ME: what is it and how it may be different from other fatigues?

CFS/ME is a long-term unexplained fatigue that has not always been present, and may occur with other symptoms such as recurrent sore throats, muscle pain, multi-joint pain, tender lymph nodes, new patterns of headaches and impaired memory or concentration. It is generally the result of major stress from perhaps a life changing event and/or an infection. ME stands for Myalgic Encephalomyelitis. Myalgia means 'painful muscles', common in many with fatigue; encephalitis is 'inflammation of the brain and nerves' - not actually detected in the strict sense in those with ME. CFS stands for Chronic Fatigue Syndrome and is well known throughout the world.

Two of the most characteristic and debilitating signs of CFS/ME are very poor stamina and delayed post-exertion fatigue. It differs from ordinary fatigue as there can be anything from hours to days between any effort and the resulting exhaustion. Repeated activity doesn't lead to improvement in strength and stamina – in fact the reverse generally happens. Sometimes the fatigue is mainly mental, and sometimes mainly physical.

* N.B. Chronic Fatigue (CFS) is used here as a generic term to cover all the names given to this syndrome including CFS/ME, CFS and Fibromyalgia (FM). Note that in some other countries, ME is almost unknown, whereas CFS is very well known.

How is it diagnosed?

Diagnosis is by exclusion of other serious illnesses and conditions when the standard blood tests come back **negative**. The physical symptoms may come under the care of different specialists, for example: endocrinologists (hormones), immunologists (infections and the immune system), neurologists (the nervous system) or gastroenterologists (the gut).

There are a number of different criteria, for example the Oxford and Canadian, which are applied to decide which type of CFS, if any, you have. Typically, the fatigue and symptoms have to have lasted for at least 6 months, be new in origin, and often need to be accompanied by 4 – 6 other symptoms from the relevant list. The severity of an individual's CFS can be measured on the an ability scale, ranging from 0 - 'Severe symptoms on a continuous basis; bed ridden constantly, unable to care for self,' up to 10 - 'No symptoms with exercise; normal activity overall; able to do house/home work full time with no difficulty.' A score of less than 2 qualifies for disability living allowance in the UK.

Who is likely to develop CFS and why?

There may be several types of people who are pre-disposed to CFS[13].

People with weak immune systems, either through damage or genetically-deficient; people who have problems detoxifying chemicals and so become sensitive to them at levels harmless to others; those with restricted diets or stressful lifestyles, e.g. shift-work, smoking etc; high achievers and perfectionists who push themselves hard and judge themselves by their results; those who constantly place the needs of others above their own and only value themselves when doing so; anxious and fearful people and those who have experienced an unresolved trauma of some sort. All these produce an on-going stress on the mind and body.

If these are the pre-dispositions to developing CFS – the time bomb ticking away, as it were - then it needs a trigger to light the fuse to precipitate CFS; some with the pre-dispositions may never develop CFS. A trigger such as a severe emotional, mental or environmental stress or a severe infection or exposure to a chemical can prove to be *the last straw*.

What mechanisms are present in CFS?

Two mechanisms may be present in virtually all those with CFS - maladaptive stress response and mitochondrial malfunction. The long

---

[13] The Optimum Health Clinic with Alex Howard and colleagues. Their very successful integrated approach includes nutrition, NLP, hypnotherapy and courses. www.freedomfromme.co.uk.

term effect of these two mechanisms may explain the array of symptoms observed.[14] [15]

Initially when we are under stress, our limbic (primitive) brain, particularly the amygdale[16], reacts (via the hypothalamus – pituitary-adrenal (H-P-A) corridor), by getting our adrenal gland to produce more adrenaline. This works fine for short-term stress, producing the primitive flight, fight or freeze reaction, after which adrenaline production drops (unless the freeze reaction gets you stuck in reacting) and eventually we return to normal. But with our modern stresses we can remain in a continuous stressful situation; our adrenal glands keep firing and start producing the stress hormones which include cortisol. Cortisol levels build up slowly and steadily producing additional fear and stress, altering our recovery time to adrenaline bursts, etc. until we 'burn out' and go into a state of high alert. Unable to sleep and produce enough cortisol to keep our mitochondria functioning, our adrenal glands stop producing their hormones. This has a negative impact on our immune system, digestive system, nervous system – in fact on every aspect of the working of our body.

The characteristics of CFS, the muscle pain of Fybromyalgia and the affects on various organs in the body could be explained by a malfunction in the mitochondria. The level of mitochondrial activity is directly proportional to the level of cortisol (controlled by nitric oxide levels) and so will be decreased during adrenal stress.

---

[14] Dr Sarah Myhill: www.drmyhill.co.uk
[15] The Optimum Health Clinic
[16] Ashak Gupta's successful approach involves retraining the amygda (part of the primitive brain) to work correctly using NLP, meditation, yoga and coaching. www.cfsrecovery.com

Mitochondria can be thought of as tiny re-chargeable power packs found in nearly every cell - effectively they are the engines of our cells, supplying the energy necessary for all cellular processes to take place.[17]

Under normal working conditions, mitochondria are the sites of energy production and house the perfect, complex cycle of chemical reactions which converts glucose (sugar) into the energy which powers the workings of our body. Given a constant supply of glucose and oxygen, the chemicals normally keep re-cycling providing us with the energy we need for our muscles, organs, body heat etc. as we need it. In the final part of energy production, ATP (adenosine tri-phosphate) is converted into ADP (-di-phosphate) + P (phosphate) and in the process releases energy for use in the body. Normally the ADP + P (+ energy from glucose) then re-combine to form ATP again, ready to release the next batch of energy. With CFS there is a problem and the cycle goes so slowly that ATP can't form in time to release the required energy, so leading to fatigue. If you carry on needing energy, your body can then break down ADP into AMP (-mono-phosphate) + P to release extra energy. AMP doesn't recycle back to ADP and so is lost to the system and is then lost to your body; this means that recyclable ATP and ADP are lost too. It takes days or weeks for the body to make ATP again from scratch which explains why 'crashes' can take so long to recover from. This shows why such approaches as Cognitive Behaviour Therapy (CBT) and graded exercise could be counterproductve.

Alternatively, energy production can get stuck in its far less efficient stage, glocolysis which doesn't use oxygen; this produces pain-causing

---

[17] Myhill, S., Booth, N.E., McLaren-Howard, J. Chronic fatigue syndrome and mitochondrial dysfunction. Int J Clin Exp Med 2009; 2: 1-16 (available to download from Dr Myhill's site: Energy; Mitochondrial failure article),

build-ups of lactic acid in the muscles (this is what happens to athletes at the end of a race but they can recover in a few minutes). Again, in CFS this recovery is a slow process – and may partly explain the pain of fibromyalgia. All in all, it appears that energy is limited in CFS due to errors in this system. This is especially noticeable in the muscles of the heart with the result that the heart can no longer pump enough energy-supplying blood around the body when a person is standing up, and can just about cope when they are lying down. CFS can, then, be thought of as a life-saver. The effect of poor blood circulation results in the shutting down of the organs in the body in a certain sequence depending on their level of priority – skin, muscles, liver and gut, brain and finally the heart, lungs and kidneys, explaining other CFS symptoms.

It is interesting to look at CFS as a protective mechanism. Initially it gets the person out of the situation which produced the stress. It also allows the body full rest. By causing a person to lie down rather than stand, it allows their heart to pump enough blood to keep their body functioning.

How is CFS treated?

As the causes and alleviation of long-term fatigue are complex, it is most important to get a correct diagnosis and understanding of the cause of your fatigue before starting most treatments.

Conventional approaches seek to diagnose a condition and then divide treatments into medical (treating physical symptoms) or psychological (dealing with the mind) to get rid of the symptoms. The medical approach helps to eliminate the symptoms by using drugs or hormones to modify the functioning of specific parts of the body; the psychological approach helps patients to recognise de-energising conscious patterns of thoughts and behaviours and then to change them (e.g. using Cognative Behaviour Therapy (CBT)). Often individuals need both approaches at the same time.

In the UK, the NHS is currently carrying out the PACE trials to test the efficacy of their psychological approach to the treatment of those with fatigue, as selected under the Oxford criteria. PACE stands for: Pacing, Activity (graded exercise) and Cognitive Behaviour Therapy: a randomised evaluation.

According to the ME Association, current conventional treatments are producing the following results:

Most people will fall into one of four groups:

- Those who manage to return to completely normal health, even though this may take a considerable period of time. The percentage falling into this category is fairly small.
- The majority, who tend to follow a fluctuating pattern with both good and bad periods of health. Relapses or exacerbations are often precipitated by infections, operations, temperature extremes or stressful events.
- A significant minority, who remain severely affected and may require a great deal of practical and social support.
- A few, who show continued deterioration, which is unusual in ME/CFS, require a detailed medical assessment to rule out other possible diagnoses.

Most complementary therapies are holistic in their approach, treating the person as a whole. Many such as Acupuncture, Reiki, Reflexology, EFT and Massage, treat various symptoms to restore the flow of energy through the body. The 'mind' approaches such as Neuro-linguistic Programming (NLP) and hypnotherapy are excellent for eliminating the cause of the problem but are not experienced at restoring the flow of energy. Hypnotherapy is used clinically to address aspects of fatigue including stress management, sleep problems, pain control and anxiety. Working as it does with the sub-conscious mind, it can be used to enhance the workings of the para-sympathetic nervous system and calm the over-activated sympathetic nervous system. Using visualisations, people can 'instruct' their body about how to start the healing process.

The links between the mind and body are starting to be discovered and more widely accepted. Psychoneuroimmunology (PNI), the study of the interaction between psychological processes and the nervous and immune systems of the human body, has produced many replicated studies that find such a link. We live in an exciting time of regular new discoveries from the multi-disciplinary approaches of PNI, Bioenergetics, Quantum Physics and Biophysics.

The most effective fatigue treatments to date have used a variety of approaches:- 'mind' therapies to re-educate the individual and the working of their body; nutrients and optimum diet to reduce environmental stresses and help the body recover; hormonal treatments to restore the correct balance and functioning of the body.

Recover your energy

Specifically, the remedy for chronic fatigue ... [and in fact, all fatigue] ... lies in the ability to tap into the unlimited natural field of energy that surrounds us at every moment.

Deepak Chopra, Boundless Energy.[18]

The most important consequence for any individual experiencing fatigue from whatever cause is that they LACK ENERGY and this has a major impact on their lives.

Until now, little has been done to address the problems of lack of energy directly. This is where the approach described in this book, *Recover Your Energy*, really takes another major step forward to assist individuals with their recovery to wellness. Based on Energetic NLP[19], which takes the best of both energy and NLP techniques to provide a powerful combination, it addresses the emotions and the beliefs behind the fatigue. *Recover your energy* provides simple methods that anyone can use for recovering, managing their own energy and accessing natural sources of energy.

These methods fit perfectly with one of the principal precepts of medicine 'first do no harm'. They can be used by an individual working on themselves and listening to their bodies; or with the guidance of a trained and skilled practitioner working with their client to help them to remove the causes for the fatigue, come up with new life strategies

---

[18] Chopra, Deepak. Boundless Energy: *The complete mind-body programme for overcoming chronic fatigue.* Rider, Ebury Publishing, 1995. Excellently presented medical examples; he applies the aurverdic approaches to health including diet, exercise and listening to your body.

[19] Art Giser, The developer of EnergeticNLP. www.energeticNLP.com

and promote optimum health and energy. The solutions come from the client rather than the therapist and so are tailor made for the individual, promoting their natural healing and empowerment.

For those with all forms of fatigue, there will be times when these practices and interventions alone will be all that is required to restore energy and health permanently. Others may not yet be at the stage to make a recovery; they may need nutritional support, hormonal treatment or an exercise programme. Whatever an individual's situation, an awareness of what has happened to their energy in the past, how they can manage it now and in the future is invaluable to the individual and practitioner.

It is important that individuals make changes to their way of thinking and to their lifestyle in order to promote recovery, otherwise regaining their energy will simply take an individual back to the original source of stress and may result in a relapse. Changes need to be made at a pace to suit the individual, devised by the individual as a result of them listening to their body and unconscious mind.

Each person's fatigue is individual to them, and the solution is often about learning about yourself, listening to yourself, and looking after yourself. Maybe, then, the name ME or 'me' is an appropriate one. The metaphor of 'putting on your own oxygen mask first', and attending to your own needs first and only then looking after others is often a very powerful healer. Otherwise you may collapse and, rather than helping others, cause even more problems! This will probably involve a whole shift in the way you think and your beliefs; remember it is, in fact, quite the opposite of being selfish. Look after yourself and then you are free to look after others if you choose or to use your skills in whatever way is most appropriate for you.

By reading this book and following the processes you can complement and enhance your existing treatments, remove your blocks to recovering your energy and learn techniques which will change your life forever for the better.

Diana Kingham 2009. www.optimiseyourlife.com.

For further detail about the discussion in this Appendix, in addition to the references above, please see:

Dr Sarah Myhill: a doctor (25 years NHS and private practice) with considerable experience of ME/CFS and other forms of fatigue. She uses a broad approach including nutritional, environmental & hormonal treatments, and offers a wide range of specialist tests. Her web-site contains a number of excellent articles and observations. www.drmyhill.co.uk

Myhill, S., Booth, N.E., McLaren-Howard, J. Chronic fatigue syndrome and mitochondrial dysfunction. Int J Clin Exp Med 2009; 2: 1-16 (available to download from Dr Myhill's site: Energy; Mitochondrial failure article),

Conclusion. 'We have demonstrated the power and usefulness of the "ATP profile" test in confirming and pin-pointing biochemical dysfunctions in people with CFS. Our observations strongly implicate mitochondrial dysfunction as the immediate cause of CFS symptoms. However, we cannot tell whether the damage to mitochondrial function is a primary effect, or a secondary effect to one or more of a number of primary conditions, for example cellular hypoxia, or oxidative stress including excessive peroxynitrite. Mitochondrial dysfunction is also associated with several other diseases and this is not surprising in view of the important role of mitochondria in almost every cell of the body, but this fact appears to have been recognised only in recent years. The observations presented here should be confirmed in a properly planned and funded study. The biochemical tests should be done on CFS patients after, as well as before, appropriate interventions and possibly on patients with other disabling fatigue conditions. It would also be good to confirm the biochemical test results in a second (perhaps government-supported) laboratory.'

UK Support groups and NHS treatment:

Action for ME   www.afme.org.uk
Association for Young People with ME www.ayme.org.uk
The ME Association www.themeassociation.org.uk
ME Support   www.mesupport.co.uk
Barts Hospital NHS CFS/ME treatment   www.bartscfsme.org
PACE: Pacing, activity (graded exercise) and cognitive behaviour therapy: a randomised evaluation. The current NHS trials for the treatment of ME and fatigue. www.thepacetrial.org

New perspectives

New Perspectives has brought together a unique set of books, for those who wish to explore how they can be the person they want to be. The objective is to offer you capability to start your own personal developmental journey around the specific area you are currently focused on, such as:

> - Improving general health
> - Recovery from illness
> - Overcoming learning difficulties
> - Moving on from long standing health problem
> - Striving to be a better parent, son or daughter
> - Building confidence
> - Reducing stress, letting go of what is no longer important
> - Improving family and business relationships
> - Better communications between yourself and others.
> - Coping with a promotion or career change
> - Setting goals and stepping up to the challenge
> - Losing anger

If you find a particular book of value for an immediate need in your life you may become curious to understand more about other aspects. We would encourage you to move to other areas that you may feel appropriate.

The books are often written by co-contributors, who are experts in their field or have firsthand experience of the topic addressed. The collaboration between the author and any contributors is crucial to the success of what they have achieved and could not be done individually – an inspirational collaboration.

The books have many stories, examples, client experiences, pictures, dialogue and sometime workbook pages to fully illustrate the point and help the reader move forward. They will be challenging. Personal change can only be achieved with commitment. Several books employ the healing power of stories that have passed down through the centuries.

As individuals grow within themselves they find that :

- Some of the daily worries of modern living melt away.
- Their focus is on the things that are really important.
- A calmer more grounded individual is less affected by negative experience, more able to cope with challenges.
- Long term illnesses change and start to shift.
- Energy and fun increase hugely.
- Inner wisdom shines through.

New Perspectives books that are currently available:

Seeing Spells Achieving
You too can 'do' health!
Recover your energy